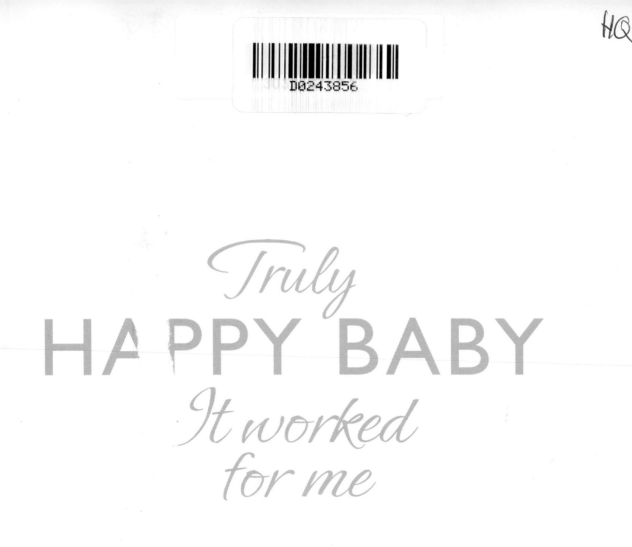

Truly
HAPPY BABY
*It worked
for me*

Thorsons
An imprint of HarperCollins*Publishers*
1 London Bridge Street
London SE1 9GF

www.harpercollins.co.uk

First published by Thorsons 2016

10 9 8 7 6 5 4 3 2 1

A catalogue record of this book is available from the British Library

ISBN 978-0-00-817252-7

Printed and bound in Spain

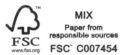

While the author has made every effort to ensure that the information contained in this book reflects NICE (National Institute for Health and Care Excellence) and NHS guidelines at the time of publication, medical knowledge is constantly changing and the application of it to particular circumstances depends on many factors. This book is intended as a reference volume only, not as a medical manual. The information given here is designed to help you make informed decisions about you and your baby, and it should be used to supplement rather than replace the advice of your doctor or other trained health professionals. Therefore it is recommended that a qualified medical specialist is always consulted for advice. The author and publishers cannot be held responsible for any errors and omissions that may be found in the text, or any actions that may be taken by a reader as a result of any reliance on the information contained in the text.

This book was awarded a Mumsnet best badge, which means the book was recommended by reviewers from the site who awarded it four stars or above.

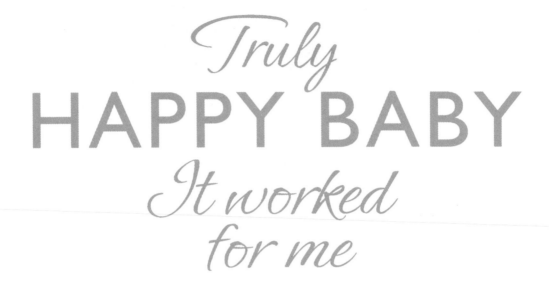

Truly
HAPPY BABY
It worked for me

HOLLY
WILLOUGHBY

with Kelly Willoughby

Thorsons

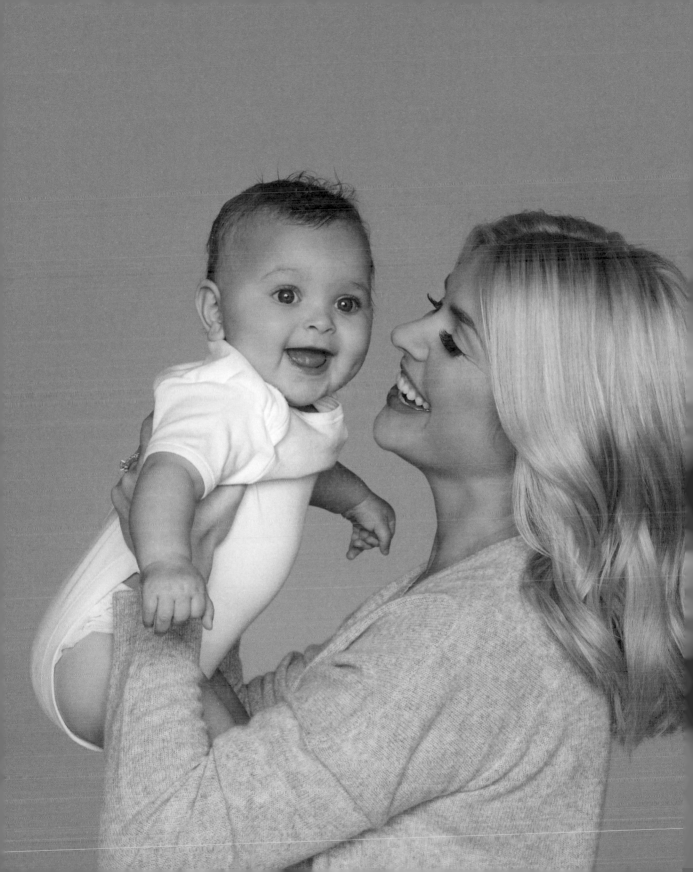

CONTENTS

So ... this is what worked for me!

I knew I would write this book when I had my first son, Harry. I couldn't believe how many times I thought – and indeed heard fellow parents say – 'Why didn't anybody tell me about this?!' There's no two ways about it, becoming a new mum or dad can be incredibly daunting. There's no other job on the planet this important where you wouldn't be given first-class training to prepare you, but as babies don't arrive with an instruction manual, this is me passing on all the things that I found worked for me, in the hope they might help you too. I've been blessed with three very different babies, so whilst I don't profess to have any official childcare qualifications (although all the advice in this book has been checked by a medical professional), I have had a lot of varied experience, coping with, and getting to know, each of my children. In this book I'll share all the best bits I've learnt along the way for how to look after my family.

The best piece of advice I can give you, and which you should try and keep at the forefront of your mind, is YOU KNOW BEST! Albert Einstein himself said, 'The only really valuable thing is intuition,' and who are we to argue with a genius?! Listen to intuition, switch off fear. When you first have a baby, you might feel bombarded with advice from friends, family and medical professionals, and some of that advice can be conflicting. This is when you have to sift through what you've been told, and then listen to you. I'm going to be really honest with you throughout this book about the decisions I made for my babies and my reasons for making them, but I can't stress enough how important it is that you go through your own thought processes, filter all the information and make the decisions that are right for you and your baby. Don't just do things because I'm saying that's what I did, and don't avoid doing things because someone else tells you not to. No one knows your child better than you, and the sooner you learn to trust and follow your gut, the more empowered, confident, relaxed and happy you will become as a parent. And, remember, no parent on the planet gets it right all the time. I certainly didn't, and more often than not the questionable decisions I made were not my own.

In this book, I've tried to give the best overview I can of the first year of your baby's life. Hopefully you'll find the more baby-led chapters such as Feeding, Sleeping and Wellbeing a really helpful but gentle guide for how to care for your baby, full of the tips that particularly worked for me. Then I've talked about Lifestyle and the changes for you and your new family, and what things you can do to make the transition smooth and the outcome even better than before. Lastly, I've tried to be as honest as I can in the Looking After You chapter, as at a time when life is so completely different, so are you, and this can feel utterly overwhelming sometimes.

It's important to say here that this isn't a rule book. One size most definitely doesn't fit all when it comes to babies so you need to spend time getting to know your baby to find out what works for you both. You might have to go through ten different soothing methods before you find one your baby likes, for example, and even then it'll probably be one you made up – see, I told you to listen to your gut! If you're at that point where nothing seems to be working and you're at your lowest ebb and most exhausted, try to remember that nothing lasts forever! You'll be in a completely different place in a month or so – just hang in there.

One final thing I should stress is that new mums don't always feel an overwhelming surge of love for their new baby when they first give birth. If that's you, you're in good company! Please don't beat yourself up about it. Just make sure you look after yourself and that little baby; you've got plenty of time to watch the love flow in – a whole lifetime in fact!

Best of luck to you and that new little baby! Let's go through this together … deep breath …

Love

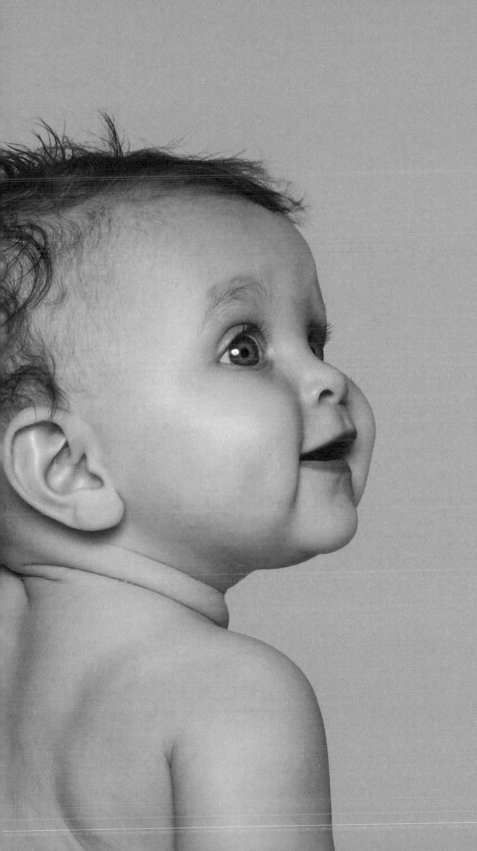

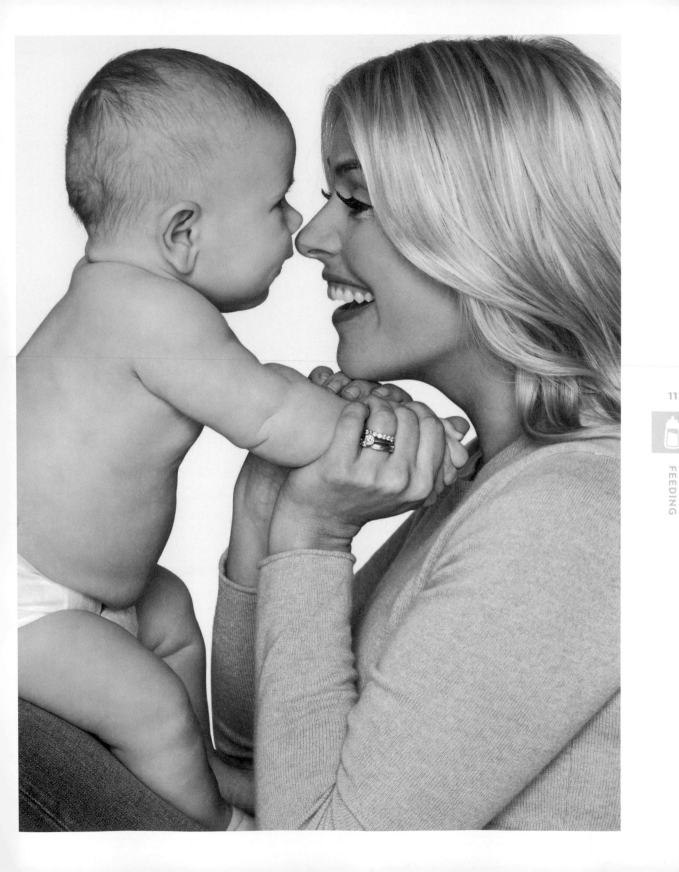

01 The need-to-knows and the know-hows

Here I've tried to give you an overview of all the paraphernalia you'll need to feed your baby – whether you're breastfeeding or bottle-feeding, or, like me, doing a bit of both. When you're trying to breastfeed, establishing your milk supply and feeding successfully can be a bit of a minefield. This section gives you a heads up on what to expect, how things change and some tips for improving your milk supply.

The only thing I would say right now, before you drive yourself crazy, is that breastfeeding doesn't always work. Even with the best will in the world and the most iron-clad determination (that I had with Chester), sometimes it's just not meant to be and you'll end up turning to formula – which is fine! All you can do is research, try everything to make it work and then see how you go. Good luck!

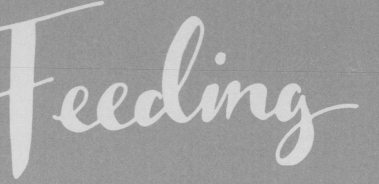

Feeding

- CHAPTER ONE -

Is it best to breastfeed rather than bottle-feed and will it come naturally?

Your new baby's finally here, and she's hungry! How you decide to feed her is ultimately your choice, because the method that's best is quite simply the one that works for you both. Breastfeeding is often described as the most natural thing in the world, but at times it can be the hardest thing to do. There's a real art to it and it's a 50/50 deal – 50 per cent you and 50 per cent your baby.

I put Harry on the breast straight away and went on to feed him successfully. However, a few hours after he was born the midwife asked me whether I'd like to top him up with a bottle so we could both get some sleep. I did this without hesitation and never had any issues putting him back on the breast. Belle arrived nearly six weeks prematurely and, despite being given drugs to slow my labour, I was expressing breast milk before she was even born! With my little reflux baby, Chester, I soon realised that sometimes no matter how hard you try, it doesn't work out. So my experience is proof that you just never know how it's going to work for you.

There's so much to consider with feeding and lots of conflicting advice! Is breast always best? Which formula should you go for? When should you wean? I hope you'll find some answers in this section that resonate with you, but ultimately – feed your baby the way you want to!

BREAST V. BOTTLE

Before embarking on this age-old debate, I want to stress that however you decide to feed your baby is right. If you're a milking machine from day dot, then lucky you! If you want to put your baby straight onto formula, then good for you. If you're hell-bent on breastfeeding, but hitting wall after wall, be at peace with giving formula! As long as you're comfortable with your decision, it's right. Feeling guilty and stressed during the first weeks of your baby's life will be far more detrimental. You'll have heard the pros and cons of both throughout your pregnancy. So, instead, I'm giving you the breast-feeding 'headlines' that convinced me to give it a go:

- Early bonding. Take it from me, when your baby opens her eyes and gazes back at you whilst feeding, you will feel an intensity like you've never known.
- Your antibodies are carried through your milk, so how could I not at least try to pass that protection on to my baby? Studies have also shown that breastfeeding has health benefits for you too.
- Breast milk evolves as your baby grows, to suit her specific nutritional needs. Although formula does contain nutrients, it stays exactly the same. Only breast milk is bespoke for your baby.
- For the lazy mum in me, breastfeeding is convenient. It's available for your baby whenever your baby needs it, there's no washing up, no sterilising and no warming a bottle in the middle of the night. So, in actual fact, for the lazy mum, once you've got it right, this could be for you!

I attempted to breastfeed all three of my babies, and I can say with brutal honesty that each time the first two weeks were very challenging. But I never give up without a fight, and with Harry and Belle I'm happy to say I was very successful. So you can imagine my frustration when with Chester no amount of grit and determination overcame the problems! I opted for bottle-feeding him expressed milk (see page 27), and eventually switched him to formula. That worked for me, so make sure you find what works for you too.

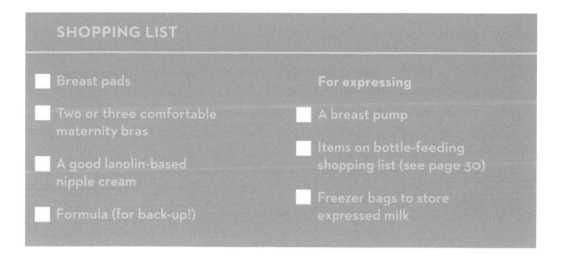

SHOPPING LIST

- ☐ Breast pads
- ☐ Two or three comfortable maternity bras
- ☐ A good lanolin-based nipple cream
- ☐ Formula (for back-up!)

For expressing

- ☐ A breast pump
- ☐ Items on bottle-feeding shopping list (see page 30)
- ☐ Freezer bags to store expressed milk

14

FEEDING

The golden nectar – colostrum ...

Before your breast milk comes in (at some point during the first two weeks after birth), your breasts produce colostrum, which is pure golden nectar to your baby. Colostrum looks a little bit like clear honey and is jam-packed with goodness for your newborn. It doesn't spurt out like milk; it's more of a slow trickle. I have to say it's hard to get your head round the fact that those few droplets are enough to stop your baby from being hungry or thirsty. Colostrum is really potent stuff, fulfilling all your baby's needs, both nutritional and functional – it's low in fats, and high in carbohydrates, protein and antibodies to help keep your baby healthy. It helps to protect your baby against infection, and also with that all-important first bowel movement – another reason new mums are really encouraged to give breastfeeding a go. Colostrum may come in before your labour even starts and, if it does, it's nothing to worry about. If anything it just means that everything is working as it should be and that your baby will be here soon! If this does happen, pop a breast pad into your bra to stop any embarrassing leaks! Breast pads will soon become your new best friend – the times I reached into my handbag for a tissue and ended up with a breast pad stuck to my palm!

Breast-milk production …

To produce good breast milk, you have to have high levels of a hormone called oxytocin – this is often referred to as the love hormone because it's triggered when you meet the love of your life! Oxytocin is needed for the let-down reflex to trigger your milk flow and can be released simply by looking at your baby, hearing another baby cry, or even just feeling warm and fuzzy. I can remember feeding Chester with the telly on in the background, and the John Lewis Christmas advert came on, the one with Monty the penguin – and I nearly flooded the place!

To have all this lovely oxytocin in your body, you have to be in love with your baby – tick! – but you also need to be well rested, well fed, not too tired and really calm and relaxed. The chances are you'll be struggling with these bits! So the best piece of advice I can give is to try to look after yourself as best you can as one thing impacts the other. If looking after yourself and your mental state means topping a screaming baby up with a bottle of formula so you can get some sleep and give your milk half a chance of coming in, then do it! If, however, you do make that decision but want ultimately to breastfeed, you should try to express off that missed breastfeed to establish your milk supply. Everyone's milk production is different. I know I had three quite different experiences with my babies.

Breastfeeding bracelets If you wear a bracelet on the arm corresponding to the breast you last fed from (so your right arm if you fed from your right breast), you'll never forget which side to use for the next feed. There are lots of lovely mummy bracelets available, or any old hair band will do – just make sure it's not too tight!

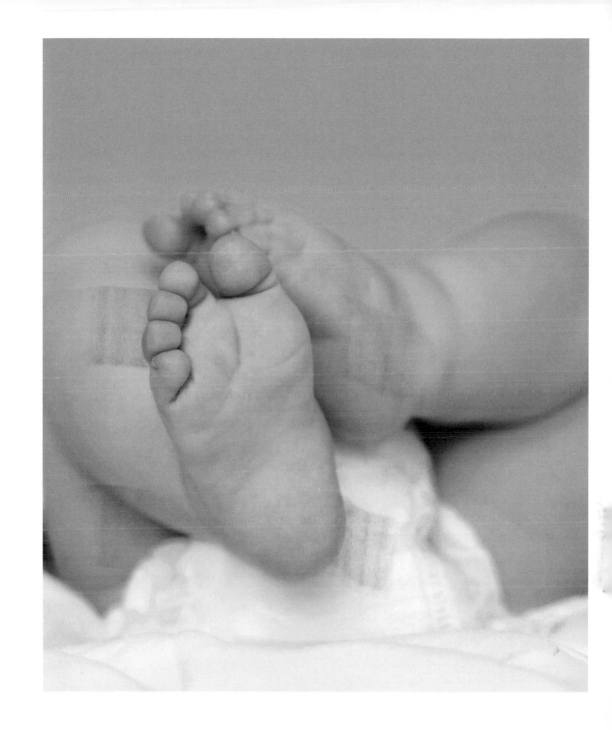

What to eat whilst breastfeeding ...

Your diet It's often difficult to keep track of mealtimes in the early weeks when you're so busy with your baby, but try not to skip meals – you need to be well nourished to produce a healthy milk supply. Now is not the time to eat less to lose weight – the old adage of making sure you get your five portions of fruit and veg a day, and a good balance of carbohydrates, protein and dairy foods, is never more important. Breastfeeding can make you extra-hungry so try to reach for a healthy snack, such as a yoghurt or some wholegrain toast, rather than the biscuit tin. These are some other foods that can help improve the quantity and quality of the milk you are producing:

- Oatmeal
- Green leafy vegetables, e.g. spinach
- Oily fish
- Lentils and pulses
- Brown rice
- Nuts and dried fruit
- Fennel and fenugreek seeds

Your baby's tastebuds How a baby reacts to your diet can vary and, whilst it's good for the baby to experience different tastes and smells through your breast milk, it's a case of trial and error. Some mums don't think twice about eating spicy foods whilst breastfeeding, as it has little or no effect on the baby, but others might find their baby really struggles to digest the milk. Some babies might show signs of lactose intolerance through mum eating a lot of dairy. If you think your baby is suffering in some way (diarrhoea, eczema, bloating, constipation, to name a few symptoms), try eliminating certain foods from your diet to see if there's an improvement. Don't overdo it on caffeine and alcohol as both can affect your baby when passed on via your milk supply.

Water I always made sure I had a large bottle of water to hand before I sat down to feed, as I'd quickly become really thirsty. It's also essential to stay hydrated when you're breastfeeding as it's very important for breast-milk production.

Cookies ... and milk! ...

A friend gave me this recipe for lactation cookies. I don't know whether it was just a placebo, but I definitely felt they made a big difference to my milk production. The magic active ingredients are brewer's yeast powder (which you can buy from all good health stores), flaxseed and some good-quality rolled oats. I've added raisins, but experiment substituting (or adding) things you love. Good flavour combinations are cranberries and white chocolate chips, and dates and walnuts.

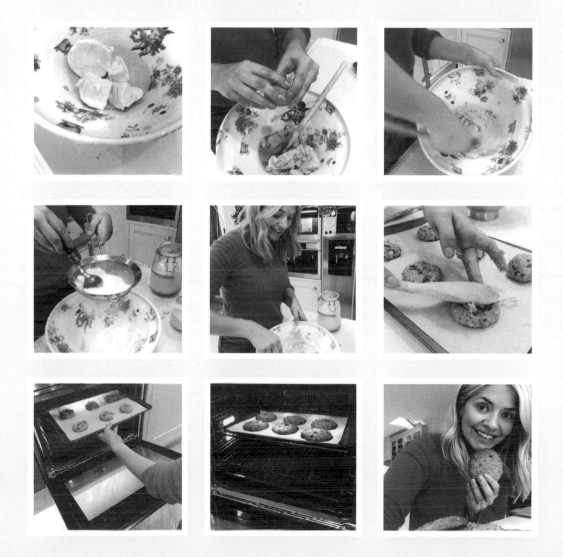

The magic ingredients

—

2 tbsp milled
  flaxseed
220g unsalted
  butter, softened
310g golden caster
  sugar
2 eggs
1 tsp vanilla extract
  or ground cinnamon
3 tbsp brewer's
  yeast powder
1 tsp salt
280g self-raising
  flour
130g rolled oats
150g raisins

—

Makes about
18 cookies

1. Preheat oven to 180°C/350°F/Gas mark 4 and line a baking sheet with greaseproof paper.

2. Mix the flaxseed and 4 tablespoons of water together in a mug and leave for about 5 minutes.

3. In a large bowl, beat together the butter and caster sugar (or use a food mixer). Add the eggs and beat in, followed by the vanilla extract or cinnamon and the flaxseed mixture.

4. In a separate bowl, sift in the brewer's yeast, salt and self-raising flour and mix together. Add this to the wet ingredients and mix well.

5. Stir in the oats and raisins (or whatever extra ingredients you've chosen), so that they're evenly dispersed through the dough. If you're using an electric mixer, you should do this part manually with a spoon.

6. Take a lump of dough (roughly a heaped dessertspoon) and, with your hands, roll into a ball. Place on the baking sheet, flattening the ball slightly with the back of a wooden spoon.

7. Repeat with the rest of the mixture, leaving a decent-size gap between the cookies because they spread as they cook. I find six balls in two rows of three work best in terms of them not sticking together.

8. Bake for 12–15 minutes, until golden. My oven produces perfect results after 14 minutes, so it's trial and error!

9. Remove from the oven and set aside for 5-10 minutes to firm up. Then transfer to a wire rack to cool completely, or dig in whilst still warm!

Switching to formula ...

You'll have been told that the official guidelines are to feed your baby solely on breast milk for the first six months. But sometimes you may decide that breastfeeding either isn't for you or isn't for your baby, and the reasons for this are broad and wide. Whatever your reason, you've got one and that's good enough for me – and it should be good enough for anybody else too (family members, midwives, health visitors, fellow mums!). Some possible reasons for calling it a day on breastfeeding are:

- **You're not making enough milk** to satisfy your baby so she's not gaining weight.
- **You've been ill** and, whether or not that ended up in a hospital stay, your milk production has lost momentum.
- **You've had mastitis** (painful engorging of the breasts – see page 69), which can sometimes lead to your milk supply drying up.
- **You're simply too tired** or overwhelmed by the breastfeeding schedule.

If you've reached this point and are feeling dreadful about it, ask yourself how many people you know who weren't breastfed. Do you think it's had a detrimental effect on their lives? The answer is likely to be ... NO! So why do we put so much pressure on ourselves? A contented baby and equally contented mummy is the most important thing, so be at peace!

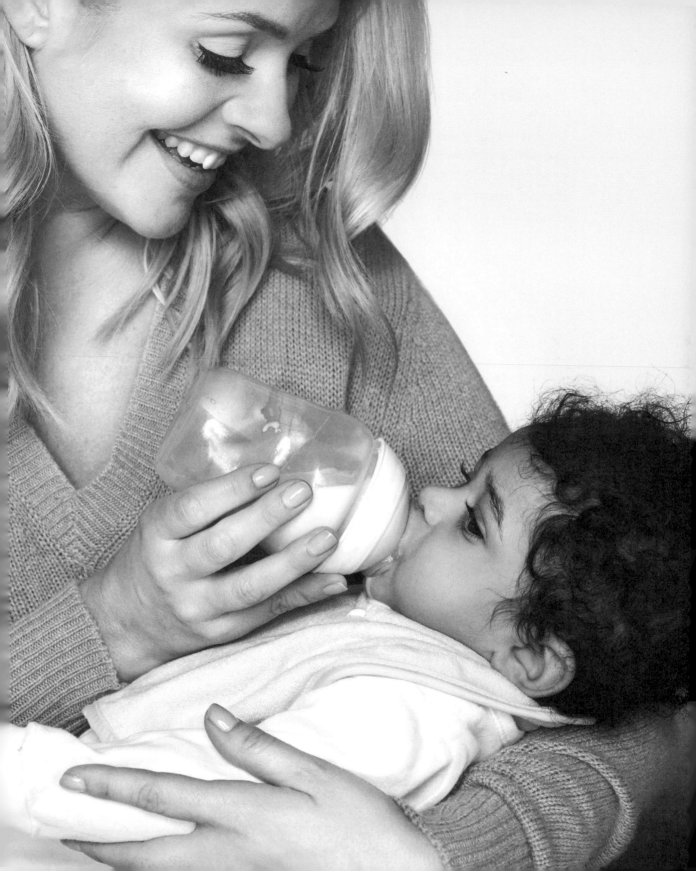

Getting it 'right' ...

It amazes me how newborns put onto the breast immediately try to latch on. It's as if they know more than you and are saying, 'Come on, Mum! I know how to do this!' Did you know that your newborn just happens to be able to see as far as the distance from your nipple to your nose, so as she is feeding your face is the clearest thing to her? And that your nipples are expanded and darkened during early motherhood so that your baby can find them easily? Mother Nature really does think of everything!

> To be able to feed your baby is a special bond, but there are plenty of other opportunities to bond – don't worry!

But, remember, no two babies are the same. You might be a milking machine for your first baby and then a complete novice with the second. Or you and your baby just might never meet in the middle. The bottom line with breastfeeding is if your baby is happy and gaining weight, you're doing it right.

To begin with, there are many things to try: where and what time to breastfeed, how to position yourself and the baby, how the baby latches on. You may be told that if you're doing it properly, breastfeeding won't hurt. Rubbish! A good friend of mine is a maternity and breastfeeding expert. Now she has her own children she feels insanely guilty that she told so many mums that it shouldn't hurt. It wasn't until she attempted to put all her advice into practice that she realised she didn't have the answers after all! Unfortunately it's always likely to hurt for the first couple of weeks, but once you've got the hang of it, it should get easier. If it doesn't, seek advice and help from your health visitor, midwife or GP. I've also covered breastfeeding issues and resolutions in the last section of this chapter (see pages 67–70).

Getting your baby to 'latch' ...

Just as every baby is different, every latch is different, but here are some pointers to help you. If your baby keeps coming off the breast or she is uncomfortable, simply try putting her on again. It does take practice.

Positioning Make sure you are comfortable (see pages 24–6) and that your baby's mouth is level with your nipple. She should be close enough to reach the nipple without straining for it, with her head and body in a straight line.

Latching To encourage your baby to open her mouth nice and wide, touch your nipple to her lips and mouth so that she can taste the milk. Then as soon as she opens her mouth, move your baby's head up and over the nipple, pushing as much of the areola in as possible. Free the bottom lip if it gets dragged in slightly to perfect the seal around the breast. The tip of the nipple should be deep inside her mouth or those strong little gums will hurt it. Don't worry about your baby not being able to breathe whilst feeding. As long as you're gently supporting her neck and shoulders and not clamping her head against your breast, she will pull away if she needs to. A good latch will mean your baby is positioned really closely against your breast.

Shaping Us mummies are all different shapes and sizes and babies only have little mouths, so you may have to forge out the perfect mouthful. To do this, hold your breast from underneath and use your thumb and fingers like pincers either side to squeeze the nipple and areola into a shape that's easier for your baby to take.

Checking the latch If your baby is latched on correctly, after a few rapid sucks she should revert to slow, rhythmic sucking, which you can watch with great satisfaction if you look at her neck as she gulps the milk down.

Seeking help Once you get the latch right, you'll never look back. If you are struggling, seek help from your health visitor or a breastfeeding organisation (see page 281). Like I said before, breastfeeding is an art – sadly, so many women give up in those early months due to lack of advice.

Breastfeeding positions to try ...

First, make sure you have plenty of cushions around you for comfort and support. Feeding can take a while, especially in these early days, so it's important you have everything you need to hand.

Try to get your baby to empty one breast before offering the second. When she is really small, she probably won't take the second, but if you've stuck to one breast, you can be more sure your baby has completed the milk cycle and taken all the nutrients she needs out of a feed. For the first few minutes on the breast your baby suckles foremilk, which is the thinner, thirst-quenching stuff, before she is hit with the fattier, richer hindmilk.

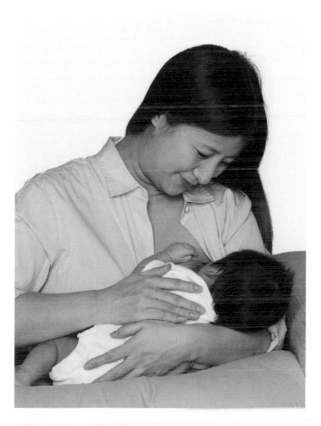

Cradle hold This is the classic breastfeeding image of a baby suckling at the breast. It's great if you can make it work as it's a relaxed and comfortable position for both of you that you can do anywhere without needing too many props! Just make sure you have a pillow under the arm the baby's head is resting on.

I used the cradle hold with Chester, and when we were struggling to feed I was advised to sit in an upright chair, place my feet on a footstool and use a breastfeeding U-shaped pillow to support him. Apparently it's the optimum feeding position and it definitely eased the strain on my back in those difficult days.

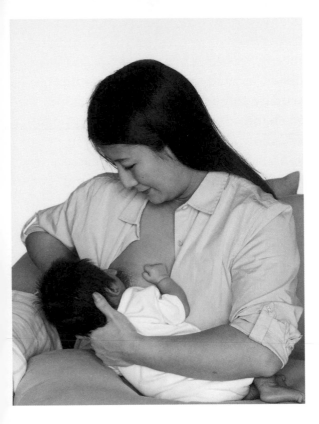

Cross cradle hold This is similar to the cradle hold but the baby's head is supported by your hand rather than in the crook of your arm. It helps if you place a pillow across your lap.

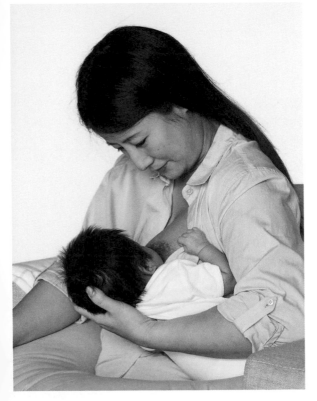

Rugby ball hold This position is particularly good for feeding twins and for breastfeeding after a Caesarean as the baby doesn't rest on your wound.

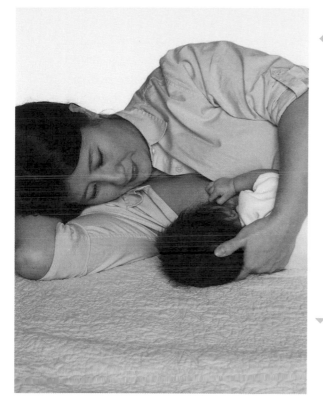

◀ Lying down on your side Lay your baby on the bed flat on the mattress and you do the same, positioning your nipple level with her mouth. You might have to lean in slightly. This is a relaxing position for both of you.

▼ Laidback hold Lay your baby on her tummy vertically along your body. Make sure she's properly latched on so she doesn't drag on the nipple.

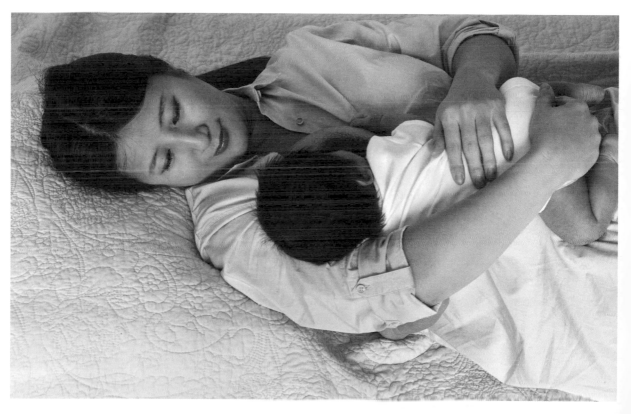

Expressing breast milk …

Expressing milk means extracting breast milk by hand or using a pump. The milk can be kept for a feed, so anyone can give it, not just you! Regular expressing is a great way to help establish your milk supply. Other good reasons to express:

- It frees you up to have a well-earned snooze.
- You might be struggling with feeding your baby directly from the breast, but still want to give her breast milk (and keep your supply up).
- Your baby might not be emptying the breast fully, so you need to express off the rest.
- You are suffering from a breast infection or engorged breasts and it's too painful to feed directly.

I expressed in different ways, for different reasons and with varying regularity, for each of my babies. In all honesty I think you need to focus on getting your milk really established for the first three months, which means looking to feed or express every three to four hours, ideally. This might sound like an arduous task at a time when you've never been so tired, but after you've put the work in your milk will be there, and more often than not it won't go away even if you want it to!

There's a lot of talk about expressing between feeds to increase your milk supply and I think it certainly helps, particularly if you're struggling with breastfeeding. If your baby is taking some milk from the breast but not emptying it, offer her a bottle of expressed milk if you have some stored – or formula – to top her up. And then express the rest of the breast to empty it fully. This way your milk will replenish and there will be plenty there for the next feed. If you are part bottle- and part breastfeeding, you might hear the term 'nipple confusion'. Personally I think this is rubbish! If you get your baby used to anything early on and keep swapping from one thing to another, she will see it as normal, but you should consider all the facts for yourself and make your own decision about this.

Due to Chester's reflux, I battled with breastfeeding for two and a half months until, eventually, I had to face the fact that breastfeeding was just not for him. He couldn't get on with it and it wasn't making him happy, which was stressing me out, which in turn was having an effect on my milk supply.

I ended up expressing every feed for the next few months until I decided that expressing, on top of sterilising and feeding with two other children in tow, was just too much and it was time to hit the formula.

If, like me with Harry, you are successfully breastfeeding all your feeds, I don't think you need to express in between, unless you want to express a bottle for your partner to give the baby so you can head to bed early and get a decent sleep! With all three of my children I expressed one of the night feeds for Dan to give so I could get to bed after the 7pm feed. But I would still wake up at around 11pm to express off that feed and save it for the following night, or else my breasts would have engorged or I'd have risked my milk not replenishing enough for the last night feed.

Breast pumps Breast pumps simulate a baby's sucking action to get your milk flowing but there are so many to choose from! I think it's better to see what your situation is before you buy a pump. When I was pregnant with Harry I googled one of those 'What to buy for your baby' lists and went shopping, and one of the things on the list was an electric breast pump. It wasn't until I actually used it that I discovered it was really noisy, which isn't ideal in the middle of the night when you've finally got the baby off to sleep. I didn't really need to express much at all with Harry, so I tried a manual hand pump instead, which was a fraction of the price, much quieter and completely portable (although it did of course take longer to express the milk).

So work out the best and cheapest expressing option for you. Mummy websites review most of the main brands and there are plenty of discussion threads. Pumps vary quite a bit in price, from the basic manual hand pump I had with Harry to hospital-grade double electric pumps. When I realised what sort of feeding regime I was in for with Chester, I rented one of these; because it was a double pump it was much quicker – and quieter – than my old shop-bought electric one.

Does expressing hurt? There's no two ways about it – when you're expressing milk you'll feel like a cow with its udders hooked up to a milking machine! But it shouldn't hurt. If you're using an electric pump there will be several power settings, and if you've got it cranked up to the highest one, hoping to produce more milk, you'll be in agony and probably produce less milk than you would if it was on a lower, more comfortable setting. Experiment to find the comfiest setting for you. If you're in pain, you won't produce the oxytocin that triggers your milk letdown (see page 15).

Another reason for expressing being painful might be the size of the part of the pump that covers the nipple. If your nipple is too big and is being squashed on all sides once you start the machine up, you might need a bigger part. There should be space around the nipple or it's naturally going to chafe, so find out if your pump has different sizes.

Once you get it right, expressing should be really easy and you'll soon find ways of clamping the cones into your breastfeeding bra so you can be hands-free to blow-dry your hair whilst pumping! Every second of you-time counts!

Storing breast milk Freshly expressed breast milk should be placed in the fridge immediately and kept for no longer than 72 hours. If you put it in freezer bags or those special milk bags and date it, you can freeze it for up to six months. Remember that breast milk changes as your baby grows and her needs evolve. If you're giving her a feed you expressed two months ago, there may not be all the nutrients she needs at that point. So if you are freezing milk, use the earliest dates first.

Milky goodness A good reason for freezing a little breast milk is that it contains natural antibodies that are good for eye infections, little cuts, etc. Even if you're not feeding any more and your milk production has stopped, you might have something in the freezer to treat your nine-month-old's conjunctivitis! (Although check with your GP first!)

SHOPPING LIST

- ☐ A bottle kit OR the items below
- ☐ 6 bottles
- ☐ 6 teats

- ☐ 1 bottle brush
- ☐ 1 steam steriliser (electric or microwave) or sterilising solution/tablets
- ☐ Washing-up liquid

If you're exclusively using formula, I'd recommend buying a formula dispenser. These are cheap to buy and usually have about three compartments so that you can measure out the right amount for each feed in advance. These dispensers are great if you are using a narrow-neck bottle, as they act like a funnel and are particularly handy when you're out and about – or if you need to make up a bottle in the middle of the night and have lost the mental ability to count scoops accurately (it happens!).

Choosing a formula ...

All the formulas contain similar stuff, but I picked one with added prebiotics. These are naturally found in breast milk and help to promote the production of friendly bacteria in your baby's gut to boost her immune system. If you find that your baby is struggling to keep her feeds down every time, it's worth trying another brand to see if it makes any difference.

Formulas suitable from birth have whey as their main ingredient as it's easy to digest and nutritionally closest to breast milk. If you find you have a very hungry baby, and one that is putting on a lot of weight due to the amount of milk she's consuming, you can get hungrier formulas, which use casein as their main ingredient. Casein is harder to digest and means that your baby won't need to feed so often, but only use this if your baby fits the profile, otherwise it can wreak havoc on your baby's digestion, which will leave you all in a pickle!

At about six months you can consider moving your baby to follow-on milk. I did because it contains extra vitamins for older babies, but there's another school of thought that says they get those vitamins from solid foods once you're weaning. Whether you choose to keep your baby on breast, infant or follow-on, don't start her on cow's milk until she's twelve months old.

Formula comes as powder that you have to make up or ready-made in cartons. Of course, the little ready-made cartons are easier and more convenient to use, but they're also a very expensive option. I always bought the big drums of powder, which I used at home, alongside a portable formula dispenser for when I was out and about. That said, there are occasions when a ready-made carton of formula is like the Holy Grail to a mum out and about! Perhaps you didn't put the lid on properly and your bottle of boiled water has leaked all over your bag; or you brought the bottles out with you, but forgot the formula dispenser. There will be at least one occasion when you find yourself running into the nearest chemist for a pricey carton of ready-made formula. And, believe me, you'll never feel more grateful for modern convenience!

How much formula to give ...

There will be feeding guidelines on the back of every formula container to help you work out the recommended amounts according to your baby's age and approximate weight. These guidelines are definitely worth considering, but crucially, don't forget that no two children are the same. They're all born at different birth weights, so, for example, the guidelines at two weeks for a baby born weighing 7lb (3kg) might not be enough food for one born weighing 10lb (4½kg). As with everything, adapt the rules to suit your baby.

Which bottle? ...

There are so many different bottles – breast-shaped bottles, anti-colic bottles, coloured bottles, glass bottles! So how do you choose the right one? Again, it's down to personal preference.

I used BPA (bisphenol A)-free bottles, which are made from food-grade plastic as opposed to one that might leak the chemical into your baby's milk. In fact, with Chester, I opted for traditional glass bottles. I know they're not to everyone's taste, but I absolutely loved them. Because I had to bottle-feed him from so young, I liked the fact he wasn't having a plastic bottle. It just felt purer to me. Apart from the risk of them getting broken, they're also quite heavy, so if your baby is intent on holding her bottle maybe opt for plastic!

I used basic bottles with Harry but tried the anti-colic bottles with Belle, and I think they're worth a whirl if you have any colic/reflux concerns (see pages 72–5). The only downside is that they have even more parts to them, so there's even more to sterilise and assemble!

Which teat? ...

Teats come in lots of different shapes, sizes and materials. It's a matter of preference but be aware you can get slow, medium or fast flow. If the hole in the teat is too big for your baby, she'll drink too quickly, leaving you in a world of winding pain! If the teat is too small, she'll have to suck really hard, which will leave her frustrated and possibly too tired to finish the bottle. There's a risk you'll mistake an exhausted baby for a satisfied sleepy one because she's had to work so hard to feed. When changing teats, give her a few feeds to get used to it, but if the milk is flooding out, you've moved up a size too early.

Bear in mind that your baby has to work harder to suck the milk from your breast than from a bottle, so it's not the change in vessel that frustrates her, it's the speed she's getting the milk. If you are combining breast and bottle, perhaps keep a slower-flow teat for longer. This will keep your baby having to work harder at the teat, so there isn't such a big difference between bottle and breast. That said, be sure she is getting enough milk and isn't frustrated.

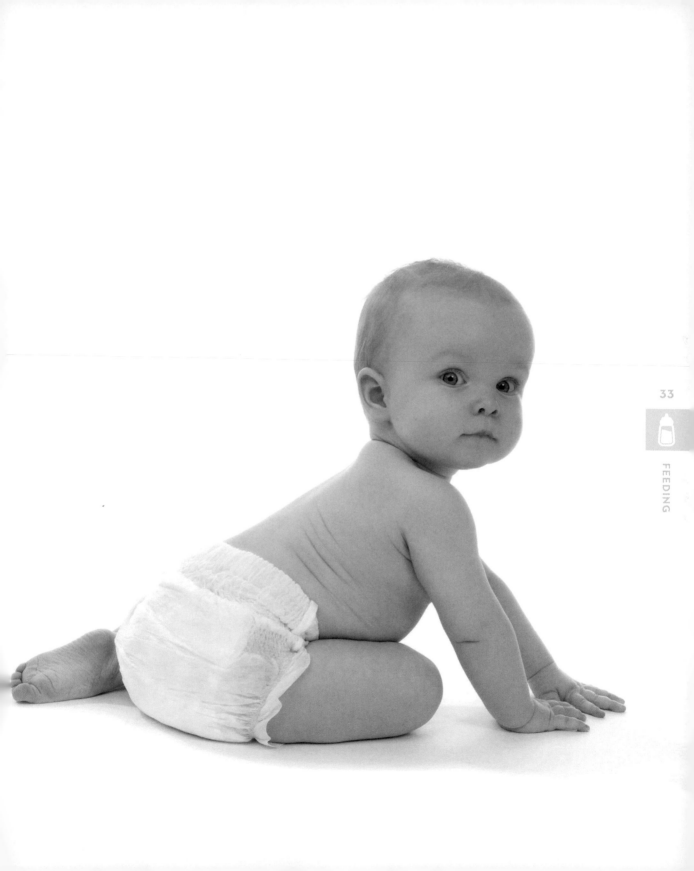

Cold or warm milk ...

The pros of cold milk It's totally up to you whether you want to warm your baby's milk before you give it to her! Some people say babies drink and digest warm milk better (and do be aware of the official guidelines - see page 38), but if yours is happy with a cold bottle then why make a rod for your own back? It's a pain in the neck if you're out and about and you suddenly have to heat a bottle for a screaming baby who's decided she's hungry half an hour earlier than you expected, especially as many cafés and restaurants won't heat milk for you for health and safety reasons. It's equally frustrating having to warm a bottle in the middle of the night. It's far easier to have ready-cooled bottles of water on your bedside table, tip in the formula from the dispenser, give it to your baby and then all go back to sleep. The less paraphernalia you need for your baby, the better!

How to warm milk If you decide to warm your baby's milk, there are numerous electric bottle warmers on the market, but in my opinion these tend to take longer to warm a bottle than standing it in a jug of boiling water. Not to mention, it's just another thing you have to find a plug socket for on the kitchen work surface!

When I asked about using a microwave to save time, I was told you can use them but it's safer not to. Microwaving doesn't evenly distribute heat through the milk, so there's a chance your baby will scald her mouth on patches of boiling liquid.

Test the temperature by tipping a few drops onto the back of your hand. If should feel just warm, not hot.

Shortcuts for warming milk I didn't warm milk for my first two children, but because Chester needed the carobel thickener (see page 73) in his milk for his reflux, I had to warm it for it to dissolve properly. Determined to make bottle-warming as hassle-free as possible, I devised a quick and easy plan once he'd moved on to formula. When I went up to bed, I would take a thermos flask of boiling water and, say he was having a 7oz bottle, I would fill a sterilised bottle with 6oz of cooled boiled water. Then when Chester needed a night feed, I would top the cooled bottle up with 1oz of boiling water from the flask, which made it the perfect temperature for the formula and carobel to dissolve and Chester to drink right away (although with carobel you do need to leave the milk to thicken for a few minutes). Likewise, during the day, say I was going out at midday for the afternoon, I'd put 7oz of freshly boiled water in a bottle, then zip it up in a bottle cosy so it would cool down slowly. By 3pm it would have cooled just enough to add the formula and be the perfect temperature for a hungry baby. But if Chester hadn't had reflux, he would have been getting room-temperature milk all day long!

Is my baby thirsty? Should I give her water? ...

I was told that, as a rule, babies get all the fluid they need from milk and shouldn't need any extra water. If it's a boiling hot day, you should feed your baby more often to stop her from becoming dehydrated.

HOW TO: BOTTLE-FEED

Whatever position works best for you, make sure you are positioned comfortably and have everything you need to hand. When you begin, your baby should make a seal around the teat with her lips to stop her swallowing too much air as she feeds. If there's milk pouring down her chin during a feed, try adjusting the position of the teat in her mouth. It should be straight, not at too much of an angle. If her lips are dragged in when you put the teat in at first, give the bottle a gentle twist to release her lips.

Your baby's head should be slightly tilted back, so there's plenty of room in her throat for the milk to flow down. If you're not holding her upright enough, it will be difficult for her to swallow freely. It's also very important that the teat is completely full with milk. Otherwise, any air in the teat will get swallowed along with the milk and you'll end up with a very windy baby on your hands.

Bottle feeding positions to try ...

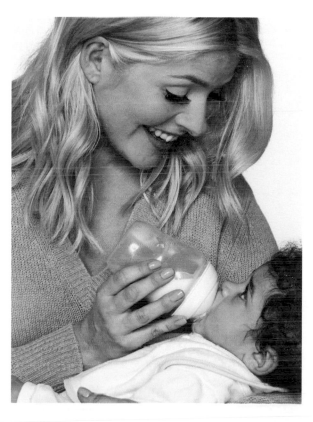

Cradle hold Hold your baby in this classic hold, where you rest her head in the bend of your arm and support her body with the rest of your arm. Her head should be positioned higher than her feet so she's slightly upright, preventing any milk from making its way into her ear and causing an ear infection. This leaves you a free hand to hold the bottle.

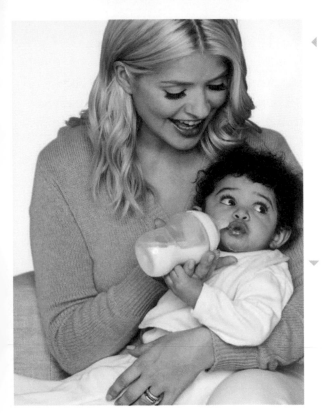

◀ Sitting-up hold Sit your baby up and lean her against your chest or rest her head in the bend of your arm. This is a great position for reflux babies and one I used a lot with Chester. It's also great for nosy babies who want to look around whilst they're feeding!

▼ The face-to-face lap hold You can do this sitting or lying. Bend your knees to make a slope and prop your baby up against your thighs, facing you. This is really nice for both of you as you can look at each other and your baby will feel fairly independent!

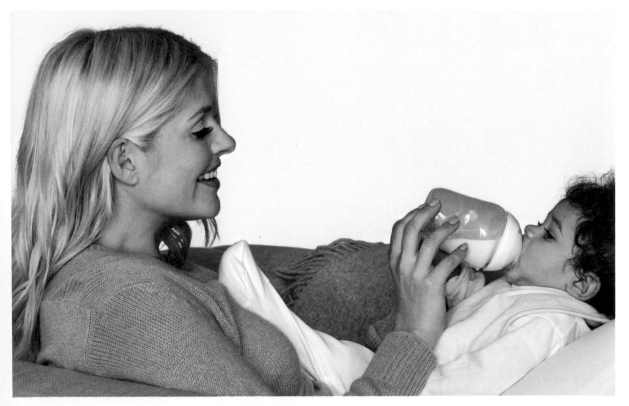

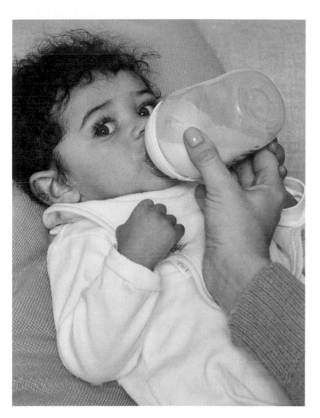

Pillow hold You don't need to always hold your baby when you bottle-feed her. If, for example, you have backache you can prop her up on a pillow and feed her that way. You can still make eye contact with her and talk to her as you feed. The only thing to bear in mind is you mustn't let her fall asleep, as this isn't a safe position for her to sleep in (see pages 91–93).

Making up formula: the rules ...

If you follow the instructions on the formula container, it will advise you to make up each bottle, one at a time, as and when you need it using the following steps:

1. Sterilise the bottle.
2. Boil the water, then let it cool for about 10 minutes before adding it to the bottle. It will still be hot. (Don't boil the water multiple times, thinking you're making it cleaner! Apparently over-boiling intensifies chemicals in the water. Think sauce reduction and how much it intensifies the flavour!)
3. Add the correct number of formula scoops to the water.
4. Cool to the perfect temperature for your baby.
5. Feed to your baby immediately.

However, I'm going to be honest with you, I didn't do it this way. This is one of those alarm-bell moments, where you need to weigh up the official advice against my experience and make your own choice. Current guidelines say you should heat the water you mix with formula to 70˚ or above to minimise the chance of any nasty bacteria forming, so while below was my preferred option, it's really up to you. If, like me, you just don't have the time or the inclination to repeat formula preparation steps 1–5 several times a day, you might find this alternative way useful.

After consulting several midwives and medical professionals about how far to take official formula advice, here's what I found out to help make life a little bit easier:

- Once sterilised, bottles will remain sterile for up to 24 hours as long as the lids are screwed on – whether you've left them empty or have put cooled boiled water in. So sterilise all your bottles for the next 24 hours in one hit, fill with the correct amount of water and pop the lids on.
- Pre-prepared bottles with only cooled boiled water in can be left at room temperature for 24 hours so you can add the formula just before you feed your baby, unless of course you give your baby warmed milk, in which case you'll have to warm the bottle (see page 34).
- You also have the option of adding the formula to completely make up the bottles after you've cooled the water, which means you have no milk to make up when your baby is hungry. If you do this, these ready-made bottles need to be refrigerated and kept cool when you're out and about, and washed and sterilised again after 24 hours whether your baby has touched them or not.
- Never save a half-drunk bottle of formula for later, otherwise you're opening your baby up to all sorts of harmful bacteria. You might feel like you're wasting so much formula but this will only happen in those early days. Soon your baby will be knocking back the whole bottle in one feeding session so there won't be any wastage at all.

The bottom line is whichever way you choose to make up bottles, you must wash, sterilise and replenish everything every 24 hours.

Washing and Sterilising ...

It's really important to wash all your feeding paraphernalia with washing-up liquid and hot water before sterilising, as sterilising doesn't do both jobs. Here's a step-by-step guide:

1. If you can, rinse bottles straight after a feed as it will save you scrubbing time at the sink later on! The best thing to get for bottles is a bottle brush. Squeeze on the washing-up liquid and make sure you get into all the nooks and crannies around the screw top and lid as well as the bottle itself.
2. Now squeeze some washing-up liquid into the teats and squidge it around, inside and out, with your fingers to make sure every millimetre is covered, then rinse the whole lot off under the tap so that there aren't any suds left.
3. After rinsing, sterilise everything.
4. You don't need to sterilise the bottle brush every time, but if your house is anything like mine, put it somewhere safe and separate to let everyone know it's for bottles only, or at some point it'll get used to scrub the grill pan!

Sterilisers I had a worktop steam steriliser for my first two babies, but I bought a microwave steriliser when I had Chester and loved it. I found it much quicker, more portable and, best of all, it didn't clutter up the kitchen worktop!

You can also get dishwashers with a special bottle-sterilising program, although I'm not sure whether I would have trusted it. It's just as easy and, to be honest, far quicker, to use a steamer steriliser than wait for a dishwasher to be full up enough to put through a cycle, and then wait another hour for it to go through. Take comfort in the fact that sterilising isn't a life sentence, although it will at times feel like you spend all your time filling and unfilling your steriliser! Once your baby reaches about six months you can switch from sterilisers to the dishwasher, but for the moment, that steriliser will become an extension of your left arm, making bottles, teats, dummies and breast-pump components safe for your baby.

HOW MUCH FOOD
IS YOUR BABY GETTING?

Breastfeeding ...

It's impossible to tell how much milk your baby is getting when you're breast-feeding. I became so obsessed about it with Chester that I started to weigh him before and after every feed, but I think that's the crazy behaviour of a mother with a reflux baby who's not putting much weight on. I didn't do that with Harry or Belle because I could see that they were gaining weight and were fine. The mistake I made with Chester was comparing the way he fed to my first two. He just didn't seem to be taking as much milk as they did, and although he was making some progress with weight he wasn't where Harry had been at that age. And there was a lesson learnt. All babies are different, and I can't say that often enough. What I really should have asked myself was: is Chester happy? Is he sleeping? Does he have plenty of wet and dirty nappies? Is he gaining weight? Does he seem content after a feed? The chances are, if you've answered yes to all those things, then your baby is getting enough to eat!

If you're worried because your baby won't settle and you think she's hungry, that's not going to help your oxytocin levels (see page 15), so seek advice from your midwife or health visitor. If you want to breastfeed and you're giving it a good go but are worried, then ask for some formula. Whatever your thoughts and concerns, just make sure you're getting all the answers that you need.

Remember: Happy, rested mummy = oxytocin = happy, sleepy baby.

Bottle-feeding ...

If you're bottle-feeding, it's easy to keep a tally of how much your baby is taking by seeing how much is left in the bottle after a feed (the same goes for if you're feeding expressed breast milk). As long as you're getting your baby weighed regularly and she's not vastly overweight or underweight, then she is getting the right amount to eat.

Baby clinic ...

You'll have various visits during the first couple of weeks from the mid-wives and then the health visitor and they'll weigh your baby. Once the visits stop you'll be issued with a PCHR red book (Personal Child Health Record), which you'll take along to a baby clinic once every few weeks or so (less frequently as your baby gets older) for your baby to be weighed and measured. The book contains percentile charts that help you to track your baby's development against the national average. There are different charts for boys and girls because they grow at different rates. The most important thing to remember about these charts is not whether your child is on the 40th or 100th percentile for weight or height, but whether she's consistently measuring around that percentile every time. There would only be cause for concern if, for example, your baby suddenly dropped from the 100th to the 40th percentile.

Early weight loss It's normal for newborns to lose up to 10 per cent of birth weight in the first week. They'll all start bouncing back by the end of the second week. Between one and four months, babies put on an average of 1.5–2lb (½–1kg) per month. By six months, babies have usually doubled their birth weight, and by twelve months it's tripled.

WINDING

Why and how often? ...

Don't be tempted not to disturb your beautiful, milk-drunk baby after a feed. If you lay her down without winding her, the chances are she'll fall asleep, but then two minutes later become a screaming, trapped-wind monster! Wind her once or twice after every feed – and if you have a really windy baby, once or twice during the feed. She will invariably let you know when she needs winding by stopping feeding and squirming slightly, or crying.

There's never a reason not to wind your baby; it can only do good. That said, if you wind her too often, and she's getting agitated because she wants to drink, perhaps you don't have such a windy baby on your hands and winding her once at the end of a feed will be enough. As with everything, once you get to know your baby, how best to wind her will become instinctive.

Little guzzlers Some babies take in too much air as they gulp down their milk, so they will probably stop halfway through, desperate for you to get the air out of their tummy. Babies might also confuse air in their tummy with feeling full and refuse the rest of a feed, meaning that they're not getting enough to eat, so make sure you give them a thorough winding.

'Muslins, muslins everywhere, on my shoulders, on my chair, everywhere.' Ha! Muslins are better than bibs because you can whip them away quickly if your baby has been sick and easily put them over your shoulder or across your lap to protect your clothing. I'd rather wash 20 muslins a day than have to get a newborn – and myself – changed every two seconds!

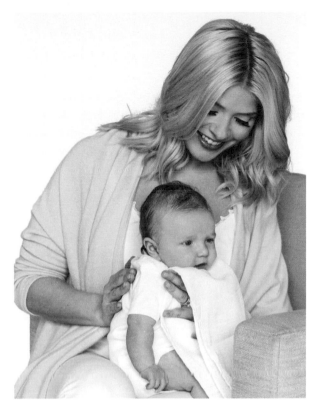

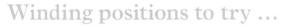

Winding positions to try ...

Classic sitting Sit your baby on your lap, support her chest with the palm of your hand, and cup her chin and neck with your thumb and fingers, whilst patting her back.

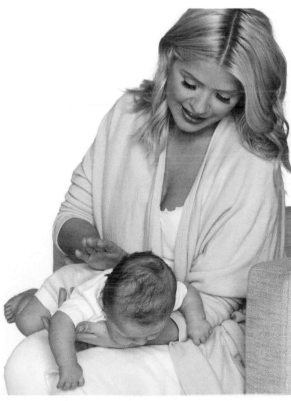

Across lap Lay your baby on your lap with her head slightly elevated and tap her back to release any wind.

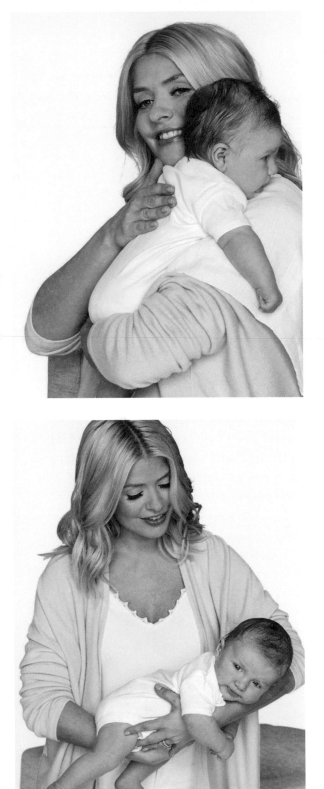

Over-the-shoulder Hold your baby over your shoulder and gently tap her back to release the wind.

Across arm Holding your baby face down across your forearm, with her head resting in the crook of your elbow, will put a slight pressure on her tummy and help to release trapped wind.

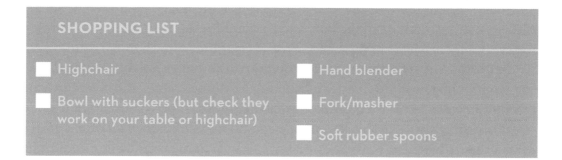

SHOPPING LIST

- ☐ Highchair
- ☐ Bowl with suckers (but check they work on your table or highchair)
- ☐ Hand blender
- ☐ Fork/masher
- ☐ Soft rubber spoons

Heat-sensitive spoons You can buy rubber spoons that are gentle on toothless gums and usefully change colour if the food is too hot!

When to wean ...

A baby's digestive system has to be mature enough to take solid food and they have to be sufficiently developed mentally (i.e. be able to hold their head up), so the guidelines are to start at six months – everything the baby needs is in breast milk until that age. However, a health professional might recommend early weaning for numerous reasons. As Chester had reflux, I was advised to wean him at about five months. Also if you have a baby who's permanently hungry and the milk just doesn't seem to be cutting it any more, starting her on a few solids may help. A sure-fire sign she is ready is if she watches you when you're eating, following the food's journey from your plate to your mouth!

Ultimately, it's up to you when to start weaning. It's lovely to finally feed your baby proper food and see all that fresh fruit and vegetable goodness going into her. This is definitely one of those situations when you know best. If you think your baby isn't satisfied by her milk intake alone, then try a little purée. But if you try it at or before six months and your baby rejects everything, perhaps it's a bit too early. Leave it, and try again a week later. Sometimes if you wean babies around other, older children, it can help them to make sense of what those solids are all about.

Head of the table …

I can't say enough about investing in a baby chair that pulls up to the table, rather than a standard highchair, so your child feels like part of the dinner party! Babies are like sponges and learn everything from their surroundings, so there's no substitute for them sitting down to meals with their family to see what you should and shouldn't do at the dinner table. Rather than you telling them not to tip their bowl all over their head, they'll soon learn it's not the done thing if they don't see anyone else doing it. Children all fidget at the table but letting them move around with food is dangerous – they could fall and choke and it makes more mess too. Sitting them at the table early on is safer and might mean they develop lovely table manners!

What worked for me …

I kicked things off with all of my children by introducing a little baby rice into their diet. I'd come down for breakfast, make up their morning bottle, pour a bit into a bowl with a couple of teaspoons of baby rice, then try feeding it to them on a spoon, interspersed with their milk from the bottle. A bit from the spoon, then a bit from the bottle and so on, just to get them used to this new texture and way of eating. Then I'd do the same at lunchtime with a little whizzed-up vegetable purée. Carrots, sweet potatoes and courgettes are all gentle flavours to start with. I didn't start them on any meat straight away, but did add fish to the vegetable purées as it's kinder on the stomach.

This all worked really well for Harry and Belle. They took to it straight away, whereas Chester insisted on doing everything all by himself. He had no interest in taking anything from the spoon I was holding, so I had to give him an extra spoon, which seemed to appease him. Another thing I did differently very early on for Chester was to try a bit of baby-led weaning. This means that you don't whizz everything up, but instead you steam a bit of carrot or broccoli and, once cooled, give it to your baby to hold, so that she's in control of holding it and putting it into her mouth. With Chester, most of it would end up on the floor but enough went in that I didn't worry and he still had milk to accompany every meal, so I wasn't concerned about him going hungry.

How to whizz! ...

If you're making up little purées, invest in a hand blender so you can cook up a carrot or two at a time and then blend and feed. You don't need one of those big all-singing, all-dancing blenders for the little portions they need at the puréeing stage. To save time and money, you may want to make up purées in batches to freeze. As they progress and grow older you can stop using the blender altogether and just mash food with a fork, then start cutting it into small bites. As you begin to introduce chunkier food, beware of choking hazards (see my warning below).

I tried to introduce lots of foods as quickly as possible. Making three different meals for three different people just isn't practical so my children, Chester in particular, have always had what we were all eating – just a whizzed-up or mashed version of it in the early stages.

Weaning warning ...

If you are giving your baby sticks of vegetables to hold, such as carrots and broccoli, steam them slightly to soften them so they're easier to bite into and digest, especially given a baby's limited number of teeth! Cut fruits such as grapes and satsuma segments into very small pieces to reduce the risk of them getting stuck in your baby's throat. I always peeled apples, too, as the skin can be tough to chew and a choking hazard. I was also told that a banana (before being mashed) is one of the most dangerous choking hazards as there's nothing to grab hold of if you need to pull it out. It's the fact that bananas are soft and break off that makes them so dangerous. As soon as your baby starts to crawl or even toddle around – you might have one who's on her feet before twelve months – don't let her move about whilst eating.

New foods and flavours ...

Ultimately you want to give your baby a varied diet and get her used to a multitude of different flavours – so before she discovers chicken nuggets (they all do!), encourage her to eat a rainbow of colourful foods. I'd suggest trying one new food at a time to make sure your baby isn't allergic to it, and introduce it with something you know she likes so she's less likely to refuse it at the first offering.

There are some brilliant ready-made foods out there and I always had a stash in the cupboard for convenience. Steaming and puréeing isn't always possible, so don't feel guilty for using them, but they are expensive compared with making homemade batches, particularly if you buy organic, which I tried to.

If at first you don't succeed! It can be frustrating to watch your baby grimace and spit out your lovingly made, delicious homemade purée, but her tastebuds are developing – what she dislikes one week might be a firm favourite the next! Portion out anything she doesn't like, label it and pop it in the freezer to try another time.

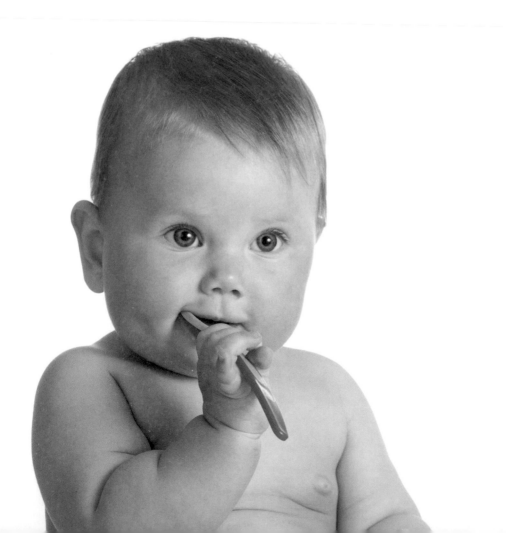

02 Milestones and routines

In this section I'm going to outline the various milestones you can expect and give you the routines I used for all my babies (which you can use in conjunction with the timetables you'll find in the Sleeping chapter – see pages 110–15). Only use them as a guide for what to expect or aim for, however, and don't get downhearted if your baby won't play ball!

Some of my children took to a routine quicker than others. It's all about having a goal and a reasonable expectation of what's achievable. The word 'routine' might suggest an exact science but, as we all know, babies dance to their own tune, so be patient. As long as you troubleshoot the reasons why your baby might not be eating much or at decent intervals and try to adapt your feeding to rectify any problems, then she will get there in the end. They all do! Tomorrow is another day and a new opportunity for your baby to form good habits.

FEEDING MILESTONES:
WHAT TO EXPECT

Very roughly (I cannot stress enough how all babies are different!), this is what you can expect over the coming months ...

First few days and weeks In the early days you'll be feeding constantly. Newborns have such little tummies that they need lots of small feeds to keep them topped up.

6 weeks–3 months During this period your little one will hopefully start having fuller feeds – hence a fuller tummy – and longer gaps between each one.

3–6 months By about three months you might start to notice your baby is really starting to respond to your gentle encouragement to get her into more of a pattern with feeding (and sleeping, as the two go hand in hand). If you only try to eke her out for an extra 5–10 minutes each feed, by the end of the day, and then the end of the week, you might find she is going a whole hour longer and eating more to boot.

6 months–1 year Once your baby reaches about six months, hopefully she'll be in some sort of routine that suits you and your family. She might not be waking for any night feeds at all and, as a result, you'll be getting the unbroken night's sleep you've been dreaming of since the end-of-pregnancy insomnia began! It's also during this time that you'll probably start moving on to weaning (see pages 46–9). Get the blender ready!

ESTABLISHING A ROUTINE

First few days and weeks: feed, feed, feed ...

I'm a big believer in feeding your baby as much as you like, as often as you like, in those first few days and weeks. You and your baby are just getting to know each other, and all that skin-to-skin contact you have whilst feeding, whether you choose to breastfeed or bottle-feed, is really nice for both of you. Breast milk, in particular, is easily digested, so it might seem in those first few days that your baby is never off the breast. But that's all good. There's plenty of time to get her into a routine. Some mums worry about snacking and that the baby is using them as a comforter or human dummy, but I say, SO WHAT! Some people seem to think that babies are born manipulative and that we need to teach them a lesson very early on to nip it in the bud, or these needy babies will go on to rule the home! Errr ... when did we become so cynical? I think we are all so concerned with how our parenting will affect our children in the long term that we forget that the most simple thing they need from the start is love, and love will get all that yummy oxytocin flowing that helps with your milk production.

Sleepy feeder Some newborns can be very sleepy, so should they be woken for a feed? I'm a bit torn on this one, as it breaks my heart to ever wake a sleeping baby, but then the arguments for feeding regularly to establish your milk supply and ensure your baby doesn't weaken are equally valid. I chose to let my babies sleep in those first couple of days and fed them when they woke up, but choose what you feel comfortable with and be guided by your midwife.

After the first day or two you'll find your baby naturally starts to wake up more often for feeds as her digestion kicks into gear. After that time, if you find she keeps falling asleep at the breast or bottle, take her socks off and tickle her toes; don't let her be too warm and snuggly. A gentle little blow of breath normally does the trick, and winding every 5–10 minutes during a feed will help too. If she is awake when she starts a feed, try to keep her awake until she finishes it or she'll never get a full feed and sleep for those coveted longer periods.

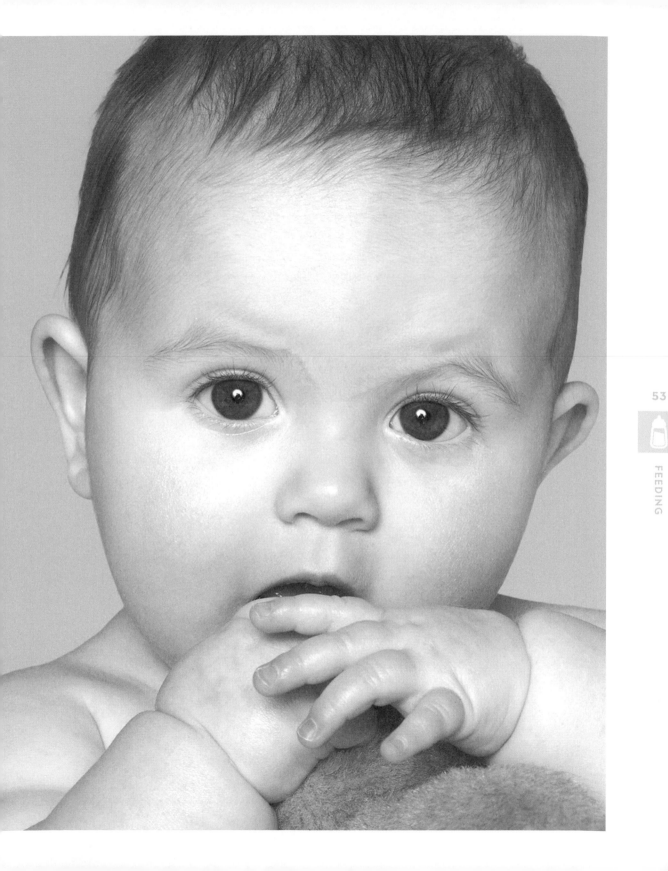

Night feeds: should you wake a sleeping baby? ...

This is probably your next question and there are two schools of thought on this:

1. Yes, do it. Filling your baby's tummy and sticking to the three-to-four-hour routine between feeds will make your baby go longer through the night, more quickly. Sometimes it's referred to as the dream feed, which you give three to four hours after you've put your baby down for the night. So this would be at around 10 or 11pm for a 7pm bedtime. It's called the dream feed because you keep all the lights off, and try to keep your baby as undisturbed as possible when you get her out of the cot. I have to say it's not easy to keep babies asleep as they invariably wake up when you start winding them before putting them back down anyway.

2. No, let her sleep for as long as she needs to. This is the only way she'll learn to stop being hungry in the night. When your baby is really little she'll probably wake up naturally for that food as her small tummy will empty quickly, but as she gets older she can sleep for longer without needing to feed. There's some research that says you go into a deep sleep after 90 minutes and will remain in that sleep pattern for the next four to six hours before you start to wake up naturally for morning. By that reckoning, if you start waking your baby up a few hours after you put her down, you risk disturbing her during her deepest sleep.

I tried both options. For me, the second option worked better – at least it did with Chester, as he learnt to sleep through from 7pm to 7am much quicker than my first two children.

I think you can only make this decision when you get to that point and know what works for you and your baby.

I always put Harry and Belle down at 7pm and did the dream feed at around 11pm. With Chester, though, because his reflux made sleeping difficult for him, I couldn't bring myself to wake him up at 11pm when he was fast asleep.

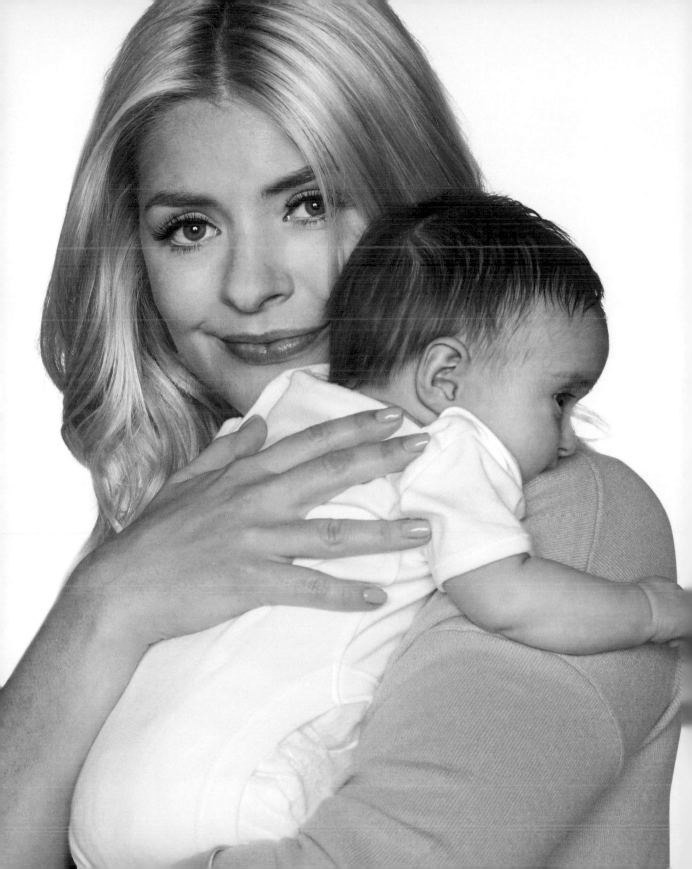

Being able to breastfeed in public gives you so much freedom. It takes a while to perfect, but once you and your baby get used to it it's the most hassle-free way to feed when you're away from home. There may be onlookers who will make you feel like you should remove yourself to the nearest mother and baby room, but I say go for it. If anyone's got an issue, it's their issue! I always had one of those breastfeeding scarves that went around my neck and then over the baby – not because I thought I was going to offend anyone, but for me breastfeeding is very personal and I just thought it was nicer for the baby to feel all snug and warm. You can get clever versions now with a semi-rigid neckline so that the material isn't across your baby's face and you can make eye contact with her.

You might not feel comfortable breastfeeding in public at first, and that's normal. It's tricky to get that latch – your baby might come on and off a few times. Then you'll get hot and bothered and think, 'Oh my God, I've got my boob out and everyone's looking at me!' And then, to add insult to injury, the oxytocin level dips, the milk slows and your baby gets even more annoyed and it's just a disaster. So go easy on yourself.

It's a good idea to have a sterilised bottle and a carton of ready-made formula with you because then you know you've got back-up. I learnt this the hard way, but once I did I never left the house without them! When Chester was about nine weeks old I took him to a fancy restaurant with some new mummy girlfriends and their babies. I thought, 'I can do this, I'm a third-time mum, I've breastfed two other children in public,' and almost felt the challenge of this somewhat empowering. Chester, however, had other plans. He screamed and thrashed about from the second we started. I ended up scurrying to the toilets to feed him, which didn't work either. I went back to the table completely mortified that I couldn't feed my child. At this point one of my mummy friends pulled a carton of formula and a bottle out of her bag and said, 'Do you want these?' I was so relieved. I pounced on them and vowed never to be caught short again.

Don't expect everything to fall into place straight away. Breastfeeding is an art!

It is possible to breastfeed and go back to work. I've done it. I've been in dressing rooms pumping milk and putting it in the fridge until I get home, and many of my colleagues have done the same. My make-up artist filled the *This Morning* fridge with her breast milk carefully labelled up so as not to confuse it with someone else's ... and so it didn't end up in Phillip's tea!

If you're lucky, you'll be able to keep up a good milk supply by expressing at regular intervals, or as best you can during your working day. If you're unlucky, your supply might start to wane, and this does happen frequently. If you are one of the unlucky ones, don't be too down on yourself. You've already done such an amazing job feeding your baby and given her a wonderful start in life. Once she sees your face come through that front door, she won't be thinking about what form her next feed takes and I imagine you'll feel the same (and probably start flooding the place before you've even said hello!).

Some of my mummy friends got into a routine of only breastfeeding the first feed of the day, and the last feed before bed. If you do this regularly enough your milk supply will respond, and even if nothing's coming in all day it will be there when you get home. It's all very clever!

ROUTINES: WHAT WORKED FOR ME

On the following pages are the routines I used for all of my babies, which I hope will be a good starting point for you and yours. A few things to bear in mind for all of them:

First, these feeding routines are all loosely based on your baby's day beginning at 7am! If it's 6am, everything will be an hour earlier – but if she wakes earlier than 6am, feed her and put her back to sleep, then start your day properly at 7am.

Second, the best way to tell whether your breastfed or formula-fed baby is getting enough milk is to monitor her weight, which you will do alongside the health visitor and by taking your baby to the health clinic for regular checks (see pages 41–2). You'll be told how often you need to go, but if your baby is gaining weight well you may only need to go once a month.

With Harry and Belle, I used to really look forward to going to see how all our hard work was paying off. There's nothing lovelier than getting a pat on the back from the clinic as they tell you how perfectly your baby is progressing. And whilst it was a different story with Chester, it was equally useful to get the reassurance and advice we both needed.

Third, there are days, even whole weeks, when your perfect baby will completely drop her routine. This is particularly common when a baby is poorly. Believe me, as soon as your baby gets the slightest snuffle, everything goes out of the window. Or she might be going through a growth spurt and suddenly need more food than normal. You need to try to work out what the reasons are and respond accordingly with either more or less food and cuddles. Just don't despair. You'll get your golden routine back in a few days, when her appetite comes back and she's not too bunged up to sleep!

Finally, I think it's a really good idea to keep a feeding and pooing diary. Sounds delightful! But seriously, for the first few weeks, day and night all roll into one so it's worth keeping a note of things – or you can now even get apps that help you keep a record of everything. Let alone what breast your baby last fed off or how much of her bottle she took, you're unlikely to remember when she last did a poo or had a wet nappy and how long she slept. Keep a record for YOU too. For example, if you're on painkillers after a Caesarean, keep a little table of when you last took tablets and when your next ones are due. You'll be amazed how four hours can slip by – you could swear you only fed two hours ago! Without keeping a record I would have been in real trouble. Baby brain and all that! Make life easier for yourself. Don't attempt to keep these sorts of things in your head!

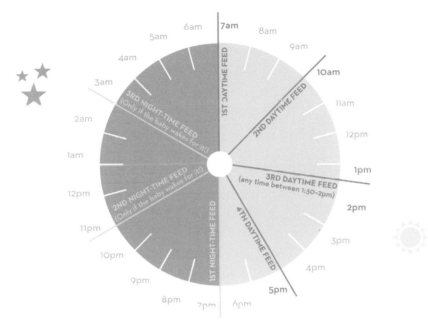

Helpful hints At this very early age, don't put pressure on yourself to stick to these times. Your baby is so young and there's plenty of time to get her into a routine. Something to bear in mind is that babies who are solely breastfed might need to feed more often than formula-fed babies, who often sleep longer between feeds. But, in general, your little one will need her little tummy fed every three to four hours.

Hungry cry Hungry cries are often accompanied by a baby clenching her fists and bringing them towards her face. A good way to tell when your baby has had enough to eat is when her hands relax and fall wide open.

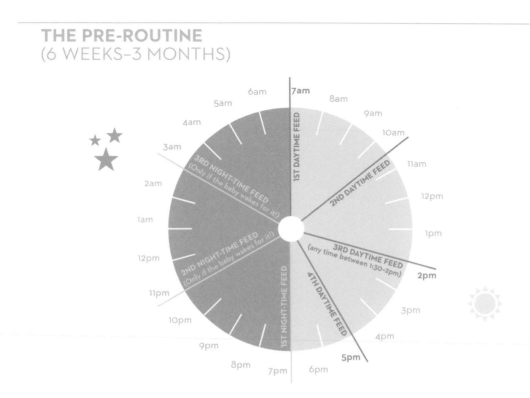

Helpful hints As the weeks go by, you're looking for your baby to go longer and longer between feeds. The first step is to try to get her to have a full feed where she empties the bottle or breast every time, so that she can last longer before she is hungry again. Then when she does feed again, she'll be hungry enough to complete the next feed so that she doesn't need to snack in between, and so on. The idea is that if your baby has had enough complete, regular feeds during the daytime, she'll get to a point where she doesn't need to wake for a feed during the night.

At this stage, your baby is still so young so, again, don't put pressure on falling into a routine. Sometimes it's tough to make your baby go longer between feeds, and the best piece of advice I can give you is that you should ask yourself a few questions, just to be sure you haven't missed anything before you feed your baby earlier than necessary. Is your baby really crying because she's hungry? Does she need a nappy change or just a cuddle? Did she have enough to eat at her last feed or is she hungry now because she fell asleep after a few minutes and you didn't wake her to finish the bottle? After the first six weeks or so, if you continue to feed your baby every time she starts to cry you'll find she only ever takes small amounts as it's more of a snack than a full feed.

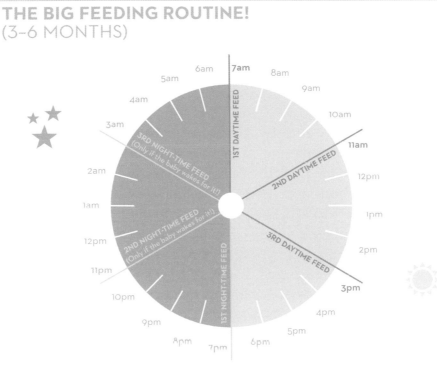

Helpful hints Since your baby arrived, you've probably been feeding her on demand, perhaps expressing some feeds or giving her formula. However you've decided to feed your baby, try to get to a point where you're leaving three to four hours between feeds. This is the way you teach your baby to fill up enough at a feed, to sleep longer between feeds and ultimately be able to sleep for long stretches through the night without needing to wake for a top-up. By the time all of mine were three months old, whether breastfed or bottle-fed, they were on a four-hourly feeding schedule, but that's just what worked for me. You'll end up forming your own schedules to suit your life. And don't be downhearted if it takes you and your baby longer to get to grips with a routine – everyone is different and that's how it should be!

Think of the four-hourly routine as a helpful framework for you to work with – if nothing else, it will give you a rough idea of when you last fed without having to keep writing it all down. It may not always work – some weeks your baby may be hungrier than others and, if you're breastfeeding, may want to cluster feed through the night. Cluster feeding is when your baby wakes for lots of feeds much closer together than usual. Young babies do this a lot, and no one really knows why. It could be your baby's way of encouraging you to produce more milk so that there's more to fill her up. This can be exhausting for you, and you'll often feel like it's never going to end and you're destined to be this feeding machine for the rest of time! Just know that it won't last forever and the good news is that it will lead to you producing oodles of milk to satisfy your baby – think how much sleep you'll both get then!

Always be guided by your baby. If you have a baby who wakes at 6am every morning, start your 24-hour clock from then. I just found that the 7am routine really worked for me. Your body gets used to a routine very quickly and you'll be shocked how you check to see what time it is and discover it's 11am or 3pm on the dot and feed time. Your body instinctively gave you a little prod. You probably won't even need to look at the clock!

One of the best things about getting my babies in a four-hourly feeding routine – in my case 7am/11am/3pm and 7pm – was it finally meant I stopped having to ask myself or Dan when I last fed the baby! Baby brain is definitely not a myth – whether it's down to all the hormones or just lack of sleep, you can have finished a feed an hour ago, and then forget immediately what time you began the last feed and completely lose track of time.

> By having a set timetable you know when the next feed is – you remember the four golden numbers 7, 11, 3 and 7!

Be adaptable The four-hour feeding routine is all about trying to find that key balance between being too flexible and not flexible enough! Being too flexible with your baby might mean you struggle to set a feeding and sleeping routine further down the line, but not being flexible enough is likely to stress you out. It's about bearing the guidelines in mind, but adapting them to suit you and your baby.

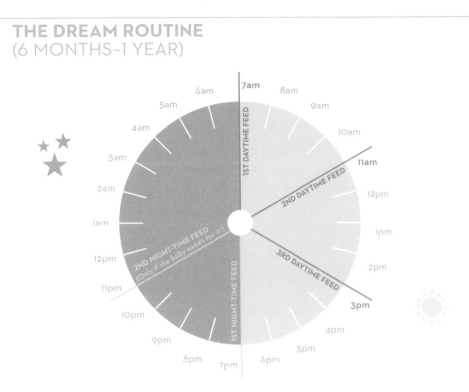

FEEDING

Helpful hints This routine will seem like a dream before you get there. An unbroken night's sleep! Perfect! Exactly your goal. Having said that, if your baby is a bit more stubborn, don't give up. She'll get there eventually and so will you. If your baby is still waking at night, don't be discouraged. Just ask yourself those troubleshooting questions I gave you in the Pre-routine Hints (see page 61) to check you're doing all the right things during the day to prepare your baby for a good night's sleep. Weaning (see pages 46–9) can help with that as solids don't get digested as quickly as liquids, keeping your baby's tummy from rumbling for longer. Whatever your situation, perhaps this little piece of information might make you feel better – or more determined to get your baby into a routine. My mum will tell anyone who will listen how I didn't sleep through the night until I was four and a half years old. Imagine that! Rather not? No, me neither! On the plus side, I can sleep for England now … or at least I could until I had babies!

Getting babies off bottles ...

By the time your baby gets to about six months old she will naturally want to start copying you, even down to the way you drink. If she reaches for your water cup, let her try to take a sip. Your baby will want to move on as much as you want her to, so be guided by her newfound interest. Give her a beaker or sippy cup with a hard spout and lid at mealtimes so she can help herself and get used to drinking out of something other than a bottle.

When your baby is getting old enough for solid food it's time to start dropping bottles. So to give you some idea, here's what I did with Chester, from about six months:

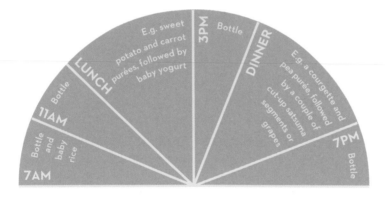

Then I gradually dropped the 11am feed, so he was just having three bottles in 24 hours. At eleven months I dropped the 3pm feed, so he was on two bottles at 7am and 7pm. At twelve months I dropped the 7am bottle and he just had a sippy cup with milk at breakfast, but be guided by what you think your baby needs all the way along. I left in that 7pm bedtime bottle for a while, as that's such a snuggly and cosy time and I really think it helped to settle him.

03 Feeding solutions

Hopefully your experience of feeding your new baby will go without a hitch, but there are a few things that can get in the way, particularly if you are breastfeeding. You might also learn that your baby has a medical reason for finding feeding tricky, such as tongue-tie or reflux, which I know all about having gone through them with Chester! These arise mostly in younger babies, and you're likely to need medical help to overcome them. In this section you'll find some of the most common issues you might face and some possible solutions to help you get on track. Never hesitate to seek the help of your GP or health visitor should you need to.

BREASTFEEDING ISSUES

Sore nipples: miracle-cure ingredient – lanolin! If your nipples are sore and raw, slather on a good lanolin cream. Tons of it! I put it on after every feed and it's honestly the only thing that helped. There is so much conflicting advice on how to treat sore nipples: everything from let them air dry, hang 'em in the wind, to putting cabbage leaves in your bra. Try these if you want to, but I always thought of chafed nipples like chapped lips and you wouldn't leave those to heal themselves in the air. Your nipples need moisturising – they need loads of lanolin cream, followed by a breast pad and bra. Another great thing is that you don't need to wash it off as it's safe for your baby. So get slathering! Sore nipples can sometimes lead to or be a symptom of other infections that may need medical treatment, though.

Infected nipples: see your GP For any infection, contact your GP. If your nipples are cracked, pink, shiny and itchy, and/or you find white spots/coating on your baby's tongue or she has an ongoing nappy rash, you might have thrush. White nipple is caused by bad blood circulation around the nipple, making it appear white, and it can be agony when your baby feeds.

Pain: try nipple shields These thin, flexible covers made of silicone act like a second skin to help reduce discomfort, and they do work. I was desperate to feed Chester but it was agony because my nipples were in such a state. Wearing a shield reduced the pain enough to get me through.

Some argue that nipple shields limit the amount of breast milk coming through, because if the baby's mouth isn't directly on the nipple, the sensation isn't there to trigger the flow. If your supply isn't brilliant shields may not be the best option as the baby will have to work really hard.

For the correct size shield, measure the diameter of your nipple. If you have a tiny baby, the tip of the largest shield may not fit into her mouth and you might need a smaller one. Equally, if the shield is too small, it won't work either. The tip of the shield should touch the roof of the baby's mouth and kick off the sucking reflex. Start with a medium size and see how you go.

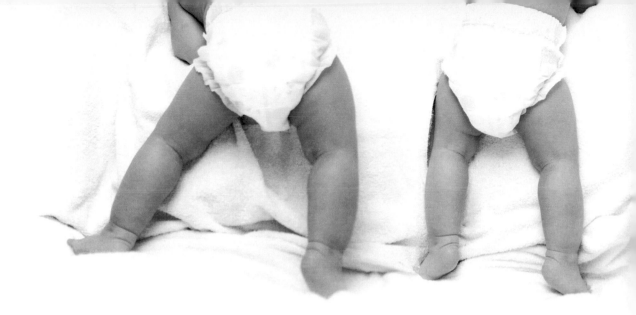

Engorged breasts: options **When** your milk first comes in (within the first two weeks after birth), your breasts might feel like they're going to explode! They will be rock solid and excruciatingly tender to the touch. All I can tell you is that it won't last for more than a week, more often only for the first 24–48 hours. As you feed (or express, if your breasts are so swollen your baby can't latch on easily), and your milk supply regulates, your breasts will become much softer and pain-free. After off-loading your milk, if you can bear it, there are other things you can do to try to reduce and relieve the pain:

- Place hot flannels on your breasts or have a hot bath.
- Try placing a pack of frozen peas on your breasts after feeding to reduce the swelling.
- Try massaging your breasts, but very gently as it will be painful.

Blocked duct: options You might develop a blocked duct in your mammary glands. The diagnosis for this is much the same as for engorged breasts, so try using heat, cold and massage. If you can face it, the best way to clear a blocked duct is to let your baby suck or to use a breast pump.

Seek medical advice! If you're really worried or finding it hard to manage the discomfort of engorged breasts and blocked ducts, seek advice from your midwife, health visitor or GP. They might advise some paracetamol for the pain, but it's best to check it's not caused by something more serious. Never wait for the fever to show up, or decide to give up breastfeeding too quickly. If it's getting you down, please see your GP. Some things just won't get better without medical intervention, so it's not worth upsetting your mental stability to let things drag on. There's always a solution.

Mastitis: immediate medical attention If you are in real agony, your breasts feel hot to touch and you feel like you've got a dose of the flu with a high temperature of more than 38°C (100.4°F), you may have a breast infection. This needs immediate medical attention. More often than not, you'll be prescribed antibiotics, but don't worry about not being able to breastfeed, as these antibiotics will be safe for your baby too – if you feel up to feeding! You may need to rely on formula for a while until the antibiotics kick in and you're pain-free enough to start feeding again. Or you may have some expressed milk in the freezer you can use in the interim. If possible, though, try to express as much milk as you can bear to, to keep up your milk supply.

If you haven't gone into labour naturally and have ended up with a planned Caesarean, your milk might take a day or so longer to come in than for someone who had a natural delivery. It's nothing to worry about, so try to be patient. If you are concerned, make sure you're asking the right questions and getting the answers you need.

If you're really worried about your baby being hungry, then this is an obvious time to ask for some formula. Why not?! As long as you put your baby on the breast for a bit (if you want to breastfeed eventually), before you top her up with formula, then you're fine. Personally, I think at no point should you feel like you have broken the sacred rule of breastfeeding by cheating with formula so early on and worry that your baby's never going to breastfeed ever again. I really think it's nonsense.

None of my babies were born by Caesarean, but my sister, whose baby was breech for the last eight weeks of her pregnancy, ended up having a planned Caesarean and experienced exactly these feelings. She really struggled with feeding, but was made to feel very guilty about giving her baby a bottle, only to discover that Lola was tongue-tied (see page 72) and their struggle was the result of many factors, rather than down to that first bottle of formula touching her lips. She says now that, looking back, had she not followed her gut feelings in the hospital and given Lola formula, they'd both have been a physical and emotional mess. So this goes to show that mum knows best and that you should listen to your instincts from the second your baby arrives. Caesarean recovery is an added stress for new mothers as they can't overdo it, so there's even more reason to reduce stress and worry where you can.

If you are breastfeeding successfully, it's important to use positions where the baby isn't putting pressure on your wound, particularly early on. The rugby ball hold (see page 25) is particularly effective.

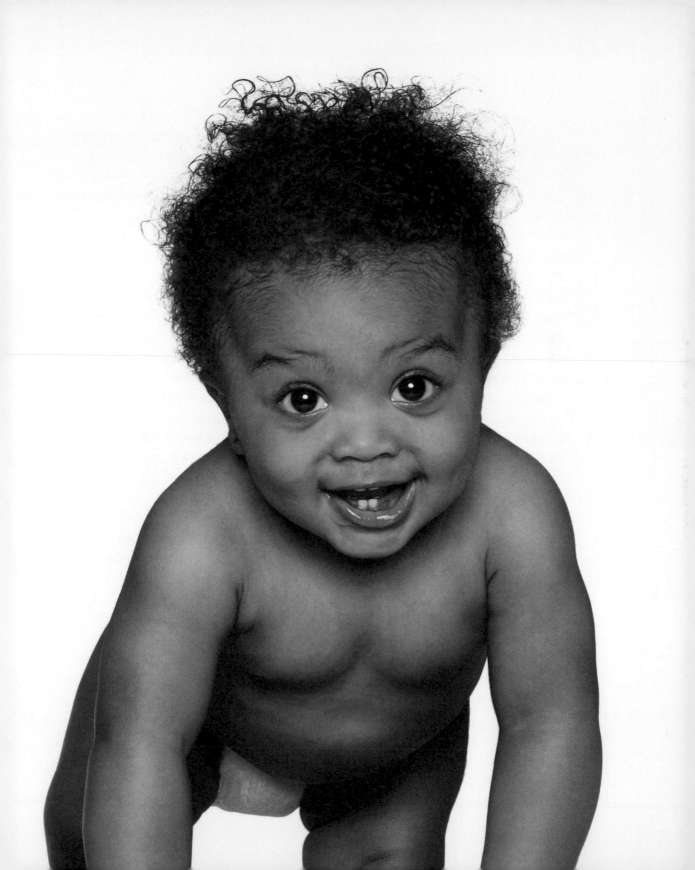

ISSUES YOUR BABY
MIGHT EXPERIENCE

Tongue-tie After two agonising weeks of trying to feed Chester and having horrific bleeding nipples, to the point where he was vomiting up my blood, I sought medical help and discovered that he was tongue-tied. This is when the tongue is restricted by a piece of tissue that isn't long or flexible enough. It can hinder a baby's latch or make it difficult for her to suck on a bottle. After discovering Chester had a tongue-tie, I realised it's not something that's automatically checked for after the delivery, so you might want to ask the question!

There's a lot of research being done into whether a tongue-tie should be cut, which I'm told is relatively pain-free. Apparently the tongue has already learnt in utero not to come forward and latch on properly, so you're trying to correct months of the baby practising in the womb and she might never get up to speed. It's up to you if you think it's worth a try. A really minor tongue-tie might snap by itself, which happened to my sister's baby.

Reflux Acid reflux is when a baby's stomach contents work their way back up the tubes and into the mouth. It can be very painful on account of the burning sensation created if the acid is strong. Lots of young babies posset when they are full, meaning they suffer from a degree of reflux, due to an underdeveloped valve that would normally keep food in the stomach. But some babies suffer worse than others and it can be very distressing for everyone.

Reflux can flare up at any point after a feed. Babies suffering it draw their legs up to their chests and cry out in pain – shrill cries that only subside when the pain has gone. Chester had silent reflux, and I'm sure he had an actual phobia of feeding at one point. It was like he was paranoid about drinking anything because he knew that as soon as he did, it was going to hit his stomach, pick up acid and come back and burn. Until I experienced it with him, to be honest I always just thought, 'Yes, all babies cry.' But reflux is a completely different situation. All the triggers for concern are there with a reflux baby: excessive crying, being sick, slow weight gain and sleepless nights.

Reflux needs medical treatment, so see your doctor straight away if you think your baby might be suffering from it. Having taken Chester to my GP, he was immediately prescribed ranitidine and lansoprazole, which treated the acid in the stomach (medicines of course change all the time, so your GP may well prescribe something else or something better).

There are many ways you can try to help your baby through it, from changing your baby's diet to trying new feeding positions. Of all these things, I would say never lay a reflux baby totally flat because it completely opens the airway, so any liquid in their system sloshes all the way up from the stomach, bringing with it acid that can burn their oesophagus. And that's what makes them cry out in pain. I used to push Chester around in the car-seat attachment on the pram base as opposed to the flat baby bassinet, as this would keep him upright and at the perfect angle to avoid discomfort. I also walked round with him strapped to me upright in a sling to keep him in the right position. Be prepared to have lots of muslins around you. Cover the sling and the car seat in muslins before you even put your baby in them. And tie your hair back, because if they can see it, they will throw up on it!

> The most crucial piece of advice I had about reflux was to keep your baby elevated at an angle at all times.

You can also give your reflux baby extra help to keep her milk down by mixing it with a thickener. After I stopped trying to feed Chester directly from the breast and started expressing, I mixed his feed with carobel, a thickening agent recommended by my GP. This kept the food weighted down, so when it hit his stomach it wouldn't so easily work its way back up. That really helped! If you are using formula, you can buy reflux-friendly formulas that already contain a thickening agent. As with all medicines and formulas, though, make sure you read and follow the manufacturer's guidelines accurately. You don't want your baby to have more than the recommended amount of anything!

Keep an eye on your diet as some food types can exacerbate the problem. If you are breastfeeding or expressing, avoid caffeine, spicy foods and acidic foods (such as fruit). Some research has also found that if you eat a lot of dairy it can have a detrimental effect. A lot of reflux can be down to a dairy intolerance, which is why cutting out dairy if you're breastfeeding might help. If you're formula feeding and you think the reflux is due to some sort of allergy, you can try lactose-free formula. This was recommended to me and I tried it but didn't notice a difference so I don't think Chester was dairy intolerant after all. Early weaning is also recommended for reflux babies – you can do it from four months.

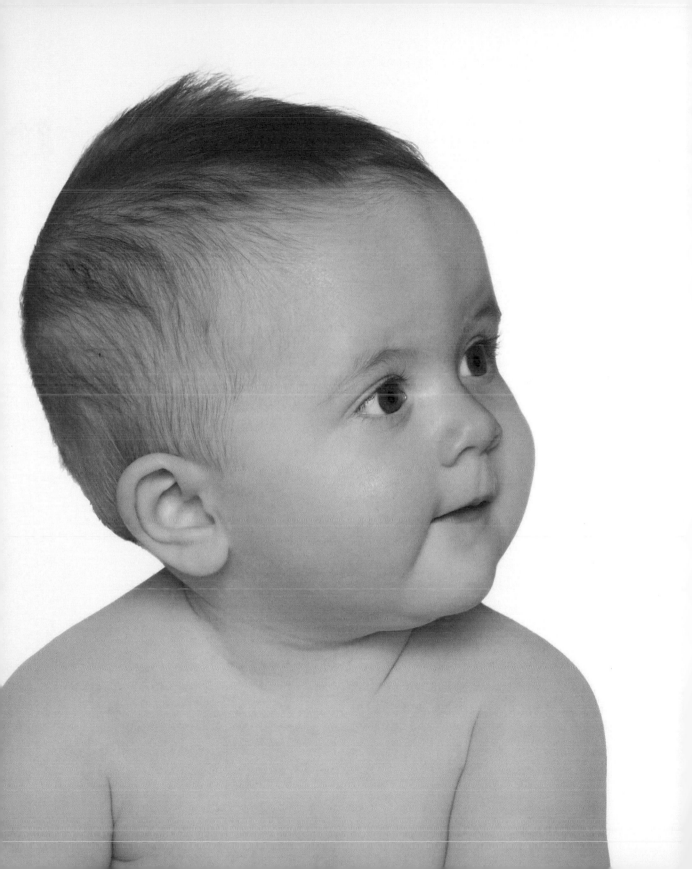

As with all these things, it's a process of elimination, so if you find something doesn't make a difference, go back to what you were doing before and try something else. To be honest, the only thing that really made a difference for Chester was the medication.

Seeing these unhappy reflux babies, who associate feeding with pain, is heartbreaking, but they will come through the other side – take it from me. If you're going through this, and feeling emotional and exhausted, try to remember that you are not alone. There's another mother in the next street going through the same! Extreme tiredness can amplify everything you're thinking and feeling, so make sure you've got plenty of support and don't bottle up the negative emotions. When I researched the timescales, I read that reflux was at its worst around four months and on the road to recovery by seven months. There is an end to it. Try some of these things and hopefully they'll make a difference to your little reflux baby. They worked for me.

Colic This is when a baby has a build-up of air or wind in her system that can make her cry for hours on end in pain. Colic and reflux have similar symptoms, but a colicky baby is content in the mornings then revs up at the end of the day.

You can buy over-the-counter remedies, including gripe water to give to your baby before every feed to try to reduce the amount of gas produced. A grandmother may suggest a glug of gripe water because in days gone by it contained alcohol. It doesn't now! Definitely don't ever give alcohol to a baby. If your baby has a severe case, the chances are that very little will help. Just cling to the knowledge that colic usually passes before a baby is four months old.

Comfort your baby as best as you can and try all the winding positions (see pages 44–5). You'll probably find your baby kicks up a stink if you even think about sitting down to calm her. She'll have you jigging and rocking her around the room, and if that's the case, get yourself out of the house. This is when you see parents driving at ridiculous o'clock, trying to settle a colicky baby and saving their backs from doing another lap carrying them around the kitchen!

Summary The subject of feeding babies is one fraught with debate about what's right, what's wrong and what to do for the best. Whether you're a breastfeeding machine, a formula fan or a mixture of the two, the simple fact of the matter is this: if your baby is happy and healthy and putting on weight, you're doing it right.

Don't get bogged down in the minutiae. It's so irrelevant, and what other people think is even more so. You know what's best for you and your baby and if you're not happy with what you're doing, then change it … Immediately.

A happy mummy means a happy baby, so there's not a moment to waste on flogging something that just isn't working for either of you. Good luck! You can do this!

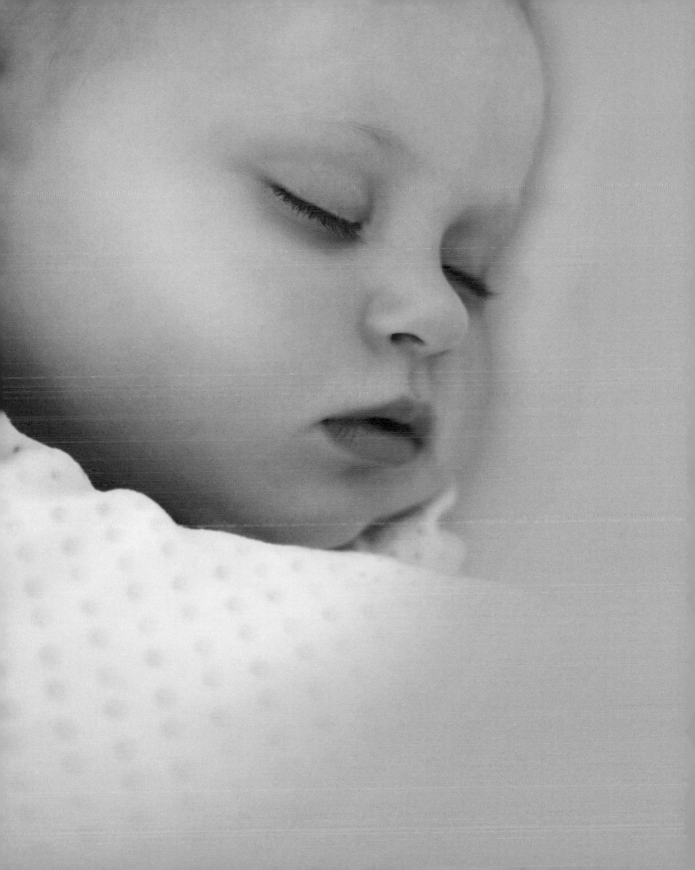

Sleeping

- CHAPTER TWO -

🌙

When will my baby sleep through the night ... so I can?!

I can't even begin to tell you how many times I've asked myself that question with all three of my children! As with much of babycare, there is a great deal of conflicting advice on how to help your baby sleep, not to mention the official government guidelines on safe sleep. So in this chapter I'm going to share with you everything I've tried and tested along the way – those things that worked for me! I'll try to give you as much information as I can about what you need and what to expect on the journey to your little one sleeping through the night.

The best piece of advice I can give you is to go with the flow for the first month or so. You will hit walls of tiredness like you've never felt before, and at times it will feel like the nights of broken sleep are never going to end, but I promise you they will. You might have to ask friends and family for help, and you might have to be strong to help your baby along in his routines, but whatever challenges you face, I promise you will come out the other side and soon forget the difficulty of those early days.

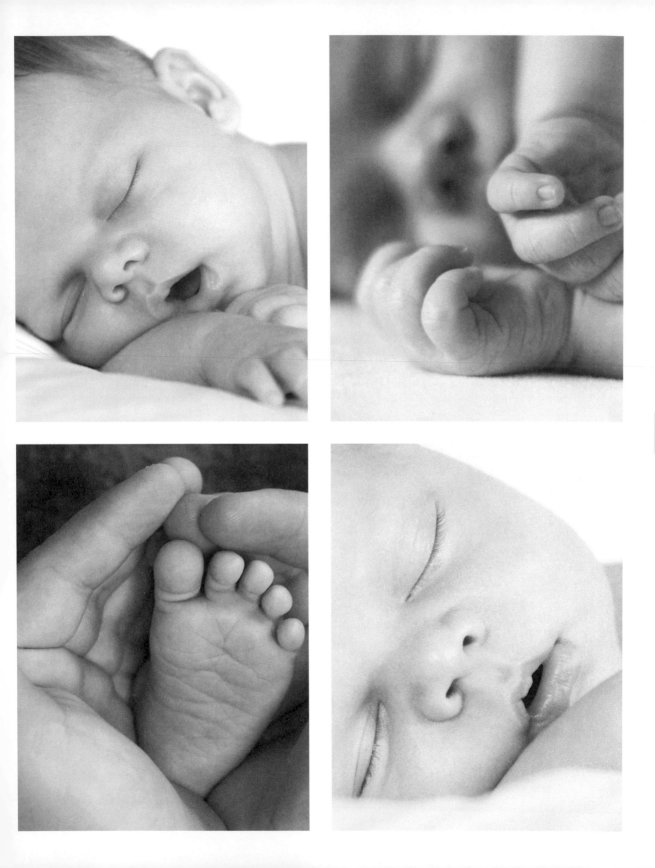

01 Making the nest

First things first – let's work out where you're going to put your baby down to sleep, how to put him down to sleep and how to create the perfect sleeping environment.

You'll be aware that you need a cot, bedding and nightwear for your baby, but you might be surprised how many options there are to choose from, and that your baby won't sleep in a cot straight away. So I've tried to pack as much practical advice as I can into this section to help you get the most out of what you buy for as long as possible, and what I found worked best for my babies (sleeping bags!).

I've also included things you might not have thought about before, such as achieving the right room temperature, and choosing a baby monitor. Like all parents, you are bound to be concerned about cot death (also known as Sudden Infant Death Syndrome or SIDS), so I've given you all the information that was passed to me on giving your baby the safest night's sleep to reduce the risks, which I hope will help to put your mind at ease.

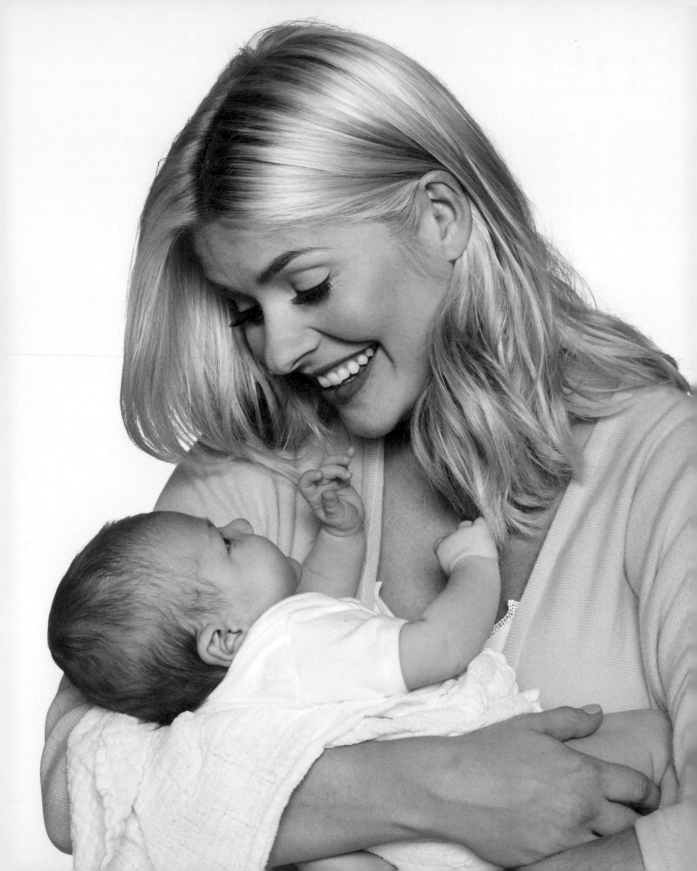

CHOOSING YOUR BABY'S BED

The early days: Moses basket and pram carrycots ...

When you bring your baby home, you will of course need somewhere to put him down to sleep. Most people start with a Moses basket – these beautiful baskets are brilliant as they enable you to carry your sleeping baby from room to room. I used the same one for all of mine, and passed it on to my sister; there's something lovely about all the babies in your family snoozing their first few months in the same basket. However, it won't feel like two minutes before your baby has outgrown it. I don't think any of mine stayed in the Moses basket for longer than two months before their little arms and legs were crying out for more space, so I would say, if the manufacture's guidance says it's suitable for overnight sleeping, use the carrycot part of your pram instead whilst you're at home in those early days. You can take it off the pram base, making it just as portable as a Moses basket, and if your baby isn't settling you can wheel him around to help him go off to sleep. Often the pram attachment is larger inside than a Moses basket, so your baby will have much more room for longer, which is great if your baby is sleeping in your bedroom and you don't have space for a cot. Another bonus is that your baby will get used to sleeping in his pram for when you do start venturing out and about.

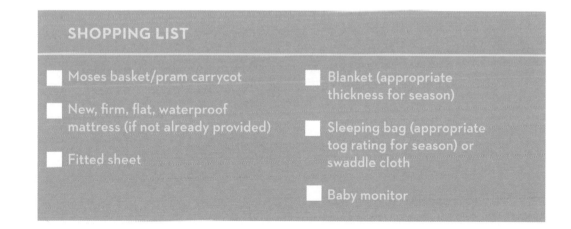

SHOPPING LIST

- [ ] Moses basket/pram carrycot
- [ ] New, firm, flat, waterproof mattress (if not already provided)
- [ ] Fitted sheet
- [ ] Blanket (appropriate thickness for season)
- [ ] Sleeping bag (appropriate tog rating for season) or swaddle cloth
- [ ] Baby monitor

Moving on: cots and cot-beds ...

When the time comes to move your baby into a cot (usually around two to three months old), a cot-bed is a great option as, when the time comes to move to a bigger bed, it'll be a much less daunting stepping stone for your baby. Cot-beds can be low to the ground, so if your toddler does fall out he will gently roll out rather than hit the floor with a thud, and another advantage is that you'll have the mattress and bedding already.

Make sure that whatever cot you buy conforms to UK industry cot safety standards. The mattress should be positioned low enough to prevent your baby rolling or climbing out and the gaps between the bars should be narrow enough to prevent you fitting a tin of baked beans through. You should also be able to adjust the height of the base as your baby grows. Once he is pulling himself up to standing, the base should be low enough that he won't fall over the top and can't climb out. However, all babies are different and some will be more determined than others to get out. If you're lucky, your baby will be more or less in the same position the next morning. Or, as happened to my sister, you'll watch in horror on the video monitor as your one-year-old pulls herself up onto the bars and drops down onto the carpet the other side ... both legs still in her sleeping bag! She was walking from ten months, so what can I tell you? Some babies are content to wait for mummy to come in and pick them up, and some try to climb Everest before they can talk!

SHOPPING LIST

- ☐ Cot/cot-bed
- ☐ New, firm, flat, waterproof cot mattress, with washable mattress cover
- ☐ Fitted cot sheets
- ☐ Cot blanket (appropriate thickness for season)
- ☐ Sleeping bag (appropriate tog rating for season)
- ☐ Comforter (like a soft toy when your baby is old enough)

WHAT (AND WHAT NOT!) TO PUT IN THE COT

Sheets and blankets ...

- **Size:** Make sure you have the correct size sheets and blankets. If you use anything that's too big, there is a risk that your baby will get tangled up in it, or if you double it up your baby could overheat. Remember, a folded blanket counts as two blankets!

- **Thickness:** You can buy special cellular blankets for babies, which have little waffle-like holes in, so your baby doesn't get too hot. Ensure these are well tucked in around the mattress and that they don't come up any higher than your baby's chest (see page 93). A baby will get too hot under a duvet so don't use them for the first year or so and never use an electric blanket.

- **Fabric:** Where possible, choose materials that breathe, such as pure cotton or bamboo. You also want to be able to put all bedding in the washing machine.

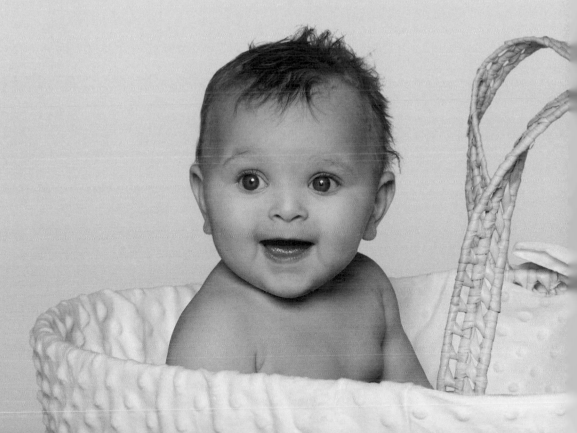

Extras ...

As a general rule, medical guidelines advise against putting anything in with a sleeping baby that could cause him to overheat, or anything he could pull over his face, causing him to suffocate.

- **Pillows:** Babies up to twelve months don't need pillows and you shouldn't put one in the cot for the same reason as above. When you do want to introduce a pillow you can get thin, anti-allergenic or temperature-control, baby-suitable ones that you can position under the sheet so your baby doesn't move it in his sleep.
- **Toys:** Don't put toys or teddies in the cot with your baby until he is at least six months old. If you do then decide to put in a toy, always be sensible about the number – don't overcrowd your baby's sleeping space.

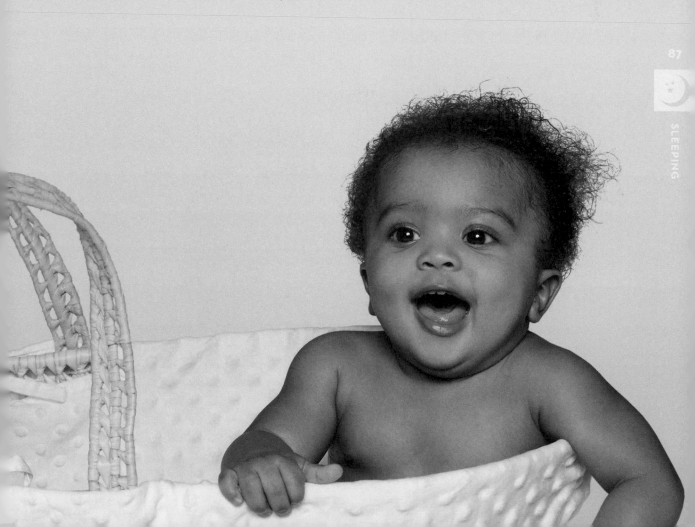

THE PERFECT BEDTIME TEMPERATURE

During the first year babies can't sweat or shiver to regulate their temperature in the same way that older children and adults can. That's why it's so important to be extra-vigilant about room temperature, particularly during the height of summer or dead of winter when there may be a significant drop or rise in temperature. Monitors that display the room temperature are brilliant for peace of mind. As a rule, the room where your baby sleeps should be 16–20°C (61–68°F), but in the table below there are some loose guidelines on adapting clothing and bedding if the temperature strays from this.

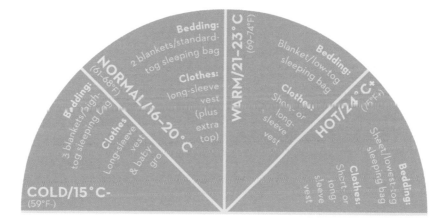

Check tummy or neck Babies always tend to have cold hands and feet, so the best way to check their temperature quickly is to feel their tummy or the back of their neck.

How to: deal with a cold room ...

If it's really cold outside, where possible set your thermostat to a constant, safe temperature or use extra blankets if the temperature dips below 16°C (61°F). Don't ever put the Moses basket or cot near a radiator or put a hot-water bottle in the cot. Equally, don't forget that if your heating is set to timed, as mine is, your baby may get cold during the night when the heating goes off. Babies don't hold the heat like we do, and can't pull the duvet up high if they wake up cold. It's all about layering, so check your baby's room temperature before you go to bed, and see whether he needs another layer.

How to: deal with a hot room ...

If your baby's room is really hot, start running a fan in one corner before bed-time to cool it down; if you hang a damp towel near the fan the evaporating water helps cool the air. Just make sure the fan is not pointing directly at the cot and that it's out of your baby's reach. Bladeless fans are great for peace of mind, but if you have a normal fan make sure it's up somewhere high, with the cable tucked away from little grabbing hands.

How to: dress your baby for bed ...

As a rule, your newborn needs to wear one more layer than you, but I'd now like to talk about something that I think is one of the greatest inventions of the modern world – the baby sleeping bag! There's a minimum weight requirement before your baby can use them, so make sure you check this first – but if he's big enough, I would definitely recommend them!

With Harry and Belle I used the original version but by the time I had Chester there was a swaddle version, where the baby's hands are also inside the bag. These are good for a baby who tends to startle himself awake. With a sleeping bag your baby will feel warm and snug whilst he's asleep without you having to worry that he's getting cold after kicking blankets off or slipping down under the covers.

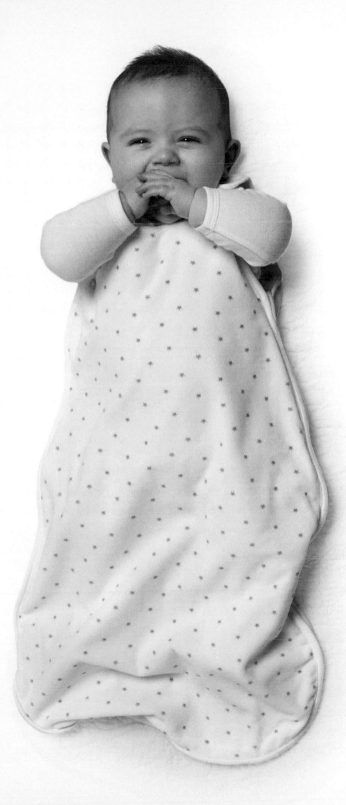

A sleeping bag fastens over the shoulders or zips at the front or side, finishing just under the chin so your baby's head can't slip down into it and risk overheating. There are different tog ratings to suit the seasons, and some come with detachable arms you can use if it's particularly cold.

I believe all of mine slept better in a sleeping bag as they felt secure without being restricted by swaddling. You have to buy bigger sizes as your baby grows, but it's not that often. Chester is using Harry's sleeping bags and there's something really lovely about that.

I think sleeping bags have revolutionised putting babies to sleep safely and comfortably. Even the action of zipping your baby into it quickly becomes a crucial part of that golden bedtime routine – as soon as you put him in it he will know it's sleepy time!

THE SAFEST NIGHT'S SLEEP FOR YOUR BABY

The threat of cot death is one of the most frightening things for a new mother to think about, but if I can say anything helpful here it's that these unexplained deaths happen to far less than even one per cent of babies and they have been on the decrease since the Back to Sleep Campaign in 1991. According to research there are several possible factors as to why this is, which I've listed below:

WHERE

- The safest place for babies to sleep is in a cot in their parent's room until they are six months old.
- Don't fall asleep with your child next to you. There is a serious risk of rolling onto the baby and suffocating him, particularly if a parent has used alcohol or drugs. The risk is significant for any newborn baby, but heightened for premature babies or those with a low birth weight.
- If your baby falls asleep in his car-seat, make regular stops to take him out of the upright position and move him to his cot as soon as possible.

HOW

- Put your baby down to sleep on his back, not on his tummy or on his side, so as not to restrict his breathing.
- Your baby should be placed feet to foot in the cot (see overleaf) – his toes should be almost touching the end of the cot to prevent him slipping down under the bedding if you're using blankets.
- Babies need to be warm but not too hot. Don't put the cot near a radiator or in direct sunlight. Don't use hot-water bottles or electric blankets. Dress your baby appropriately for the season and room temperature, but never use hats or head coverings.

WITH

- You should have a firm mattress with a waterproof cover, and bedding should be kept to a minimum (depending on temperature), tucked in well either side of the mattress. Don't use a duvet, which could end up covering the baby's head.

- Don't put pillows or soft toys in the cot. These all put your baby at unnecessary risk of suffocation.
- Don't smoke during pregnancy or expose your baby to tobacco smoke after birth. Until the effects of vaping are known, treat e-cigarettes with the same caution.
- If you use a sling, don't curl your baby up in it. You should also always be able to see his face easily when glancing down.

Baby monitors ...

There are several types of baby monitor to choose from. I had the most basic audio monitor for Harry and Belle, which did the job perfectly. However, when it was time to put Chester in his own room I invested in a video monitor so I could see if there was any obvious reason for his crying, beyond the reflux – and, I have to say, I'm a convert! I was really anti video monitors when they first came out. I worried I might become addicted to staring at my sleeping baby on a screen, but having now tried it I love it! And it's not just for when they're little. My sister has always had a video monitor for my niece, Lola, and says they're even more useful when your baby gets older, particularly when they make the move from a cot to a bed. You can check what he's up to, without having to go up for a peek and risk him playing up just to get you to come back up after the lights are out.

If you choose a video monitor, you may be tempted to stand the camera part on the edge of the cot to get the best close-up picture of what's happening, but this is dangerous. It's much safer not to have such a close-up view, and to put the camera high up above the cot, keeping the hazardous cable out of reach of your growing, grabby baby – if he pulls out the cable, one end is connected to the mains and there is also a danger that it might get caught around his neck.

Audio monitors with breathing sensors You can get audio monitors with breathing-sensor pads that you place under the cot mattress. I used one of these for Chester because of his reflux, but didn't feel it was necessary for either of the other two.

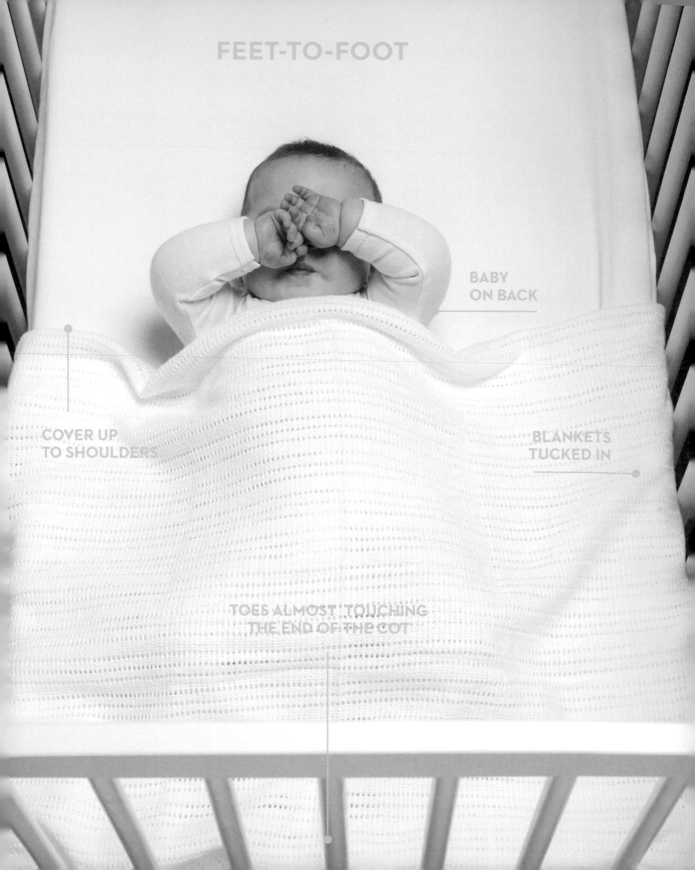

DECISIONS FOR YOUR INTUITION TO MAKE

Moving your baby to his own room ...

There will come a time when you're comfortable enough to move your baby to his own bedroom. It's just one of those things you have to weigh up and do when it feels right for you, although the official guidelines say not to do it before your baby is six months old.

Some parents find it hard moving their baby into a separate room, but I found having a baby monitor, especially the video monitor, made it feel like they were by my side without actually physically having them there. Once they were in their own room I noticed they slept better and for longer periods without being disturbed by me or Dan. I would always say goodnight and then close the door. If they get to the age where they ask you not to shut the door any more, then fine, but as a baby I think they're in their own peaceful little place.

Elevating the cot ...

If your baby has reflux, try elevating the cot slightly at the top end. This worked with Chester as it meant he wasn't lying flat, which helped prevent the acid in his tummy coming back up to burn his throat. It can also help your baby to breathe better if he has a cold. Your baby's feet should be in the correct position at the end of the cot, so there's no risk of them wriggling down – just make sure the cot elevation isn't too steep.

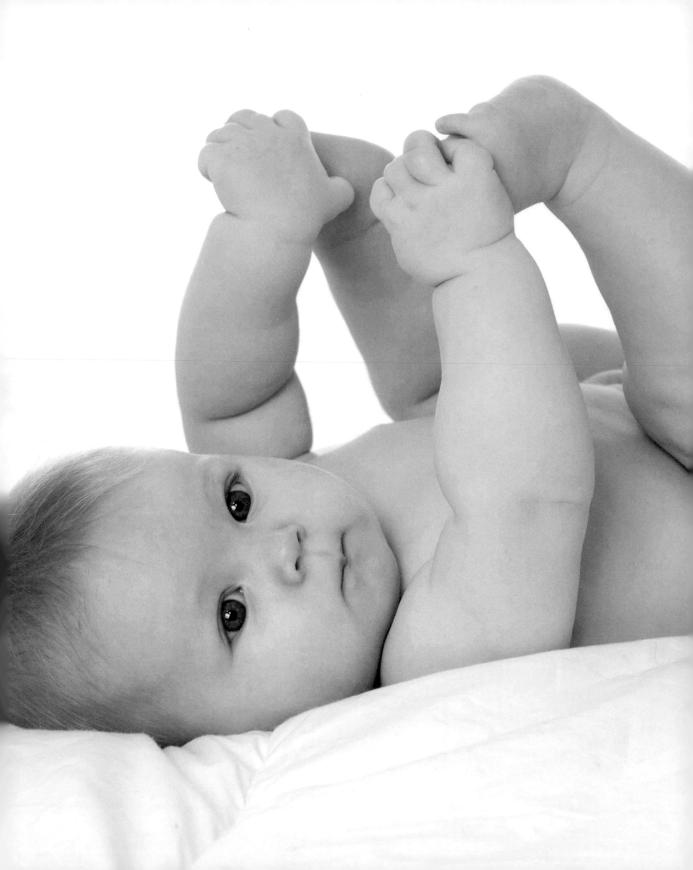

Chester wasn't a baby who could sleep, feed, then sleep. It took me an hour to feed him, an hour to wind him, then I'd have to keep him upright long enough for the acid to calm down. Moving around the house at night to feed him and disturbing the rest of the family wasn't an option.

Co-sleeping ...

In my mind, co-sleeping, which means sleeping with your baby in your bed, is never a good idea as the risks completely outweigh the advantages. That said, there are now bedside cots on the market that butt right up to the bed, making you feel like you're sleeping with your baby, without any safety risks – I had one with Chester and loved it. In the first week or so we were sort of co-sleeping, but with a divide between us that I could roll down and roll up so it was safe to do. It was really nice to have him next to me in those early days and made feeding much easier, particularly as he had a tough start due to the reflux, which meant that feeding and settling him at night took a long time!

As soon as Chester's reflux became more serious, he and I moved onto the sofabed in the lounge, so I could be near to the kitchen and away from the rest of the family trying to sleep peacefully upstairs. He just wasn't able to be that baby who sleeps, feeds and then sleeps. It took me hours to feed and settle him back to sleep, then he'd be waking soon after to start the whole process again. Dan was back at work and Harry and Belle were at school and needed their sleep, so moving downstairs was the only option that worked for me and that particular baby.

02 Milestones and routines

When it comes to milestones and routines, cling to this fact: there is no such thing as 'the norm' when it comes to babies! They are all completely different and do everything at different speeds, but in an attempt to give you a rough idea of what to expect, I'm giving you my experience.

So, whilst you were pregnant, you did all your research and now that your beautiful baby is finally here you're wondering when's the best time to get him into a routine. It's quite simple – not now! Relax! Don't even think about planning when your baby is and isn't going to sleep. You can have memorised every sleep plan you've ever read about, but none of this will be of any use to you until your baby is at least two months old – and even that's early! It's certainly a good idea to have all those sleep goals and ideals at the back of your mind, and I know I read everything I could get my hands on and had aspirations for how to train the perfect baby – but believe me when I say that for the first few days and weeks of a baby's life, he is in charge, so take your lead from him and listen to his needs.

HOW MUCH SHOULD YOUR BABY SLEEP?

Sometimes it can be reassuring to see things in black and white, but before you look at the diagrams below you should be aware that it is perfectly fine for your baby to sleep more or less than the hours given, regardless of age. Every baby is different, and it's important not to tie yourself up in knots about what your baby is or isn't doing compared with the national average!

Newborns will sleep for about two-thirds of the day and make no real distinction between day and night, so you'll both be in a 24-hour cycle of eating and sleeping. As the months go by and your baby becomes more alert, he will naturally reduce the number of hours he sleeps during the daytime and increase the hours he is sleeping through the night, which is exactly what you want to achieve.

AVERAGE BABY SLEEP CYCLES

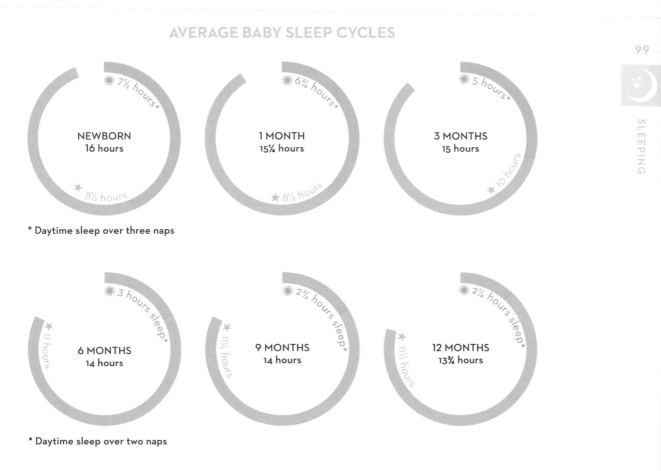

NEWBORN
16 hours
☀ 7½ hours*
★ 8½ hours

1 MONTH
15¼ hours
☀ 6¾ hours*
★ 8½ hours

3 MONTHS
15 hours
☀ 5 hours*
★ 10 hours

* Daytime sleep over three naps

6 MONTHS
14 hours
☀ 3 hours sleep*
★ 11 hours

9 MONTHS
14 hours
☀ 2¾ hours sleep*
★ 11¼ hours

12 MONTHS
13¾ hours
☀ 2¼ hours sleep*
★ 11½ hours

* Daytime sleep over two naps

The diagrams on the previous page give you a rough estimate of your baby's sleep patterns, but here's how this all translates into real life and what you can expect at the different phases of development.

First few days Let your baby feed and sleep on demand. I fed on demand around the clock with all my babies. At this stage I don't think you can put them on the breast too much. As soon as my baby had gone to sleep I'd grab forty winks myself. You'd be amazed how much benefit you get from those little power naps – enough to recharge you for the next cycle of feeding, pooping and sleeping.

3–6 weeks If your baby is eating well, you might notice that he's sleeping for slightly longer stretches. You might find that feeding every three hours is sufficient, so if your baby has woken up at around 7am, you'll be following a 7am, 10am, 1pm, 4pm, 7pm schedule. If your baby is getting a full feed every time, without snacking in between, he will be on track for sleeping longer at night.

6 weeks–3 months It's the time spent asleep during the daytime that is reduced. Harry started to sleep for only about an hour in the morning, when it had previously been one to two hours.

3–6 months We all know the golden goal of a baby sleeping through the night, and in this next period you might just experience it! Yes, I know, a pipe dream come true! What you're trying to achieve is your baby sleeping for about three hours during the day and up to eight hours at night. It's also around this time you might decide to move your baby out of his Moses basket or pram carrycot – I remember putting mine down in their big cot for the first time and thinking how teeny tiny they looked, but if you spend time getting them used to it they'll take to it just fine.

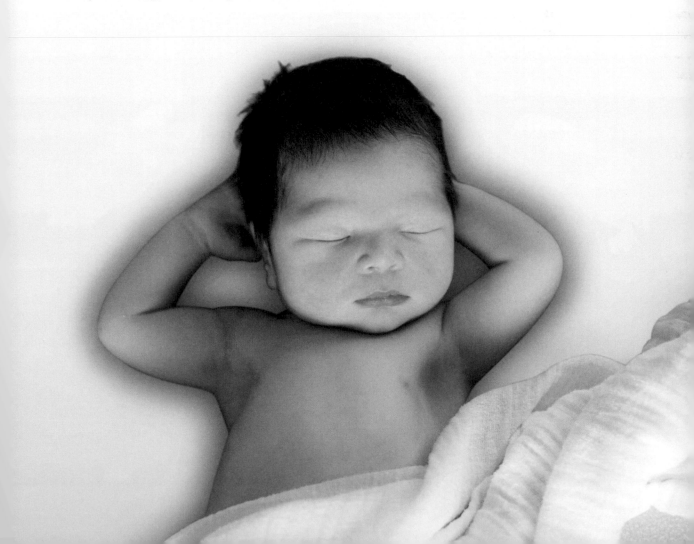 6 months–1 year By about six months your baby will be having a morning snooze, a long lunchtime sleep and an afternoon nap. The first of these to go is the afternoon nap, followed by the morning one, and soon your baby will only be having one main sleep a day after lunch. You should be getting more sleep too as your baby is probably in his own room at night.

As you near the end of your baby's first year, he may be sleeping through from about 7pm until at least 6am. How exciting is that?! It's not to say that you won't have the odd sleepless night – due to illness, maybe, or sometimes your baby will just wake for no apparent reason. Maybe it's his little mind working overtime to reach the next developmental milestone. Who knows?! Just know that there's no feeling like the first time your baby sleeps through and you'll all get there. I promise!

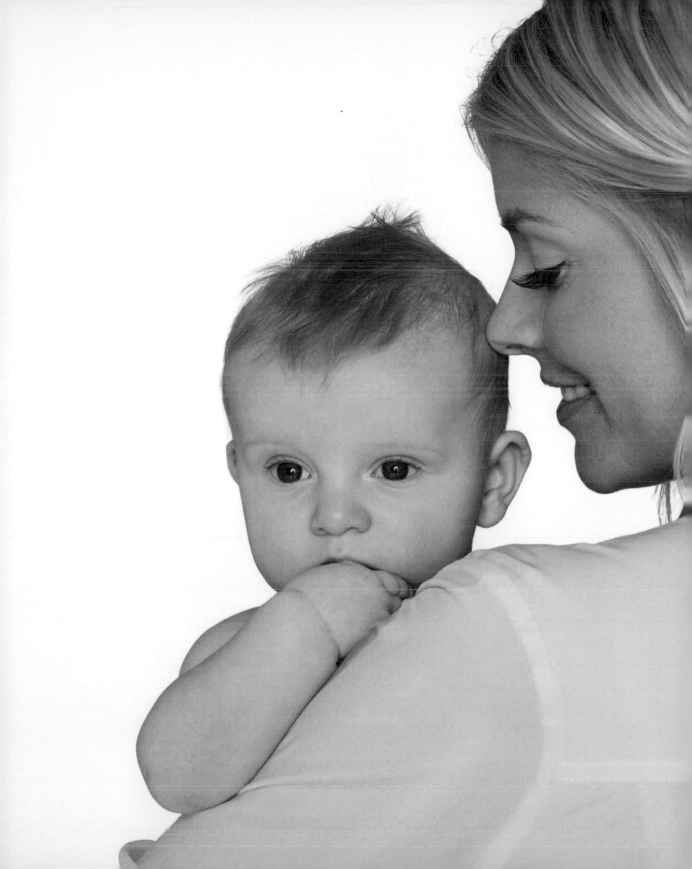

ESTABLISHING A ROUTINE

The first 24 hours: routine? No chance! …

No matter what your birth experience, you're likely to feel completely exhausted yet euphoric. That euphoria will give you the energy you need for what's to come – but it's not the time to start thinking about routines! There is a school of thought that recommends waking your baby every two or three hours to get him used to feeding regularly and to kick-start your milk supply. But I think if you are expressing regularly and your baby isn't screaming for food, then why wake him? The only time I would agree with waking him for a feed is if he's born jaundiced or prematurely and is very tiny and weak. Then it is important to get advice from your midwife and other healthcare professionals.

But with that in mind, I can't talk about sleeping without talking about feeding. A full, satisfied baby sleeps … well, like a baby! Milk is sleep juice. Remember, the more of this you can get into your baby, the longer he is going to sleep; and the more he sleeps, the happier he is and the hungrier he will be when he wakes up; and the more he'll eat when he wakes up, the longer he will sleep – and the happy cycle goes on.

I can remember being surprised at how awake all of mine were just after they were born. But after that first feed all your baby will want to do for the first 24 hours or so is sleep. Seize your chance to sleep and recover together. After the initial feed you'll find your baby might go hours before waking for another feed. Let him sleep and wake up refreshed and fully charged to have a big, alert feed next time, otherwise he'll just keep falling asleep and you'll wonder whether or not that last feed actually counted.

Depending on your milk situation, you might want to express milk your baby has missed to encourage your supply, or hand express any colostrum and keep it for when your baby wakes up. It's so important to get some of your strength back, so if your healthy baby gives you the opportunity to get your head down, then sleep! He will soon let you know if he's hungry.

Warm feet If newborns have warm feet, they sleep better. I would always put their bedtime babygro on with their socks on top. Always! If you feel a baby's feet, they're always cold, even if their hands are warm.

Your baby knows when he feels hungry and tired, so be guided by him. It's the only way this is going to work and, as a new mother, is the only thing you instinctively know how to do. Feed him on demand, cuddle him, sing to him, shhh him, pat him, rock him, soothe him, but, most of all, love him. It's what you're there for, and if you get that right, your baby will be happy, satisfied and secure, and the golden sleep routine you so desire should follow.

Once your baby has woken up to the new world around him, you'll find you don't have to wake him for a feed at all. His tummy will let him know when he's hungry and he'll let you know. It is a wonderful feeling to see your satisfied, milk-drunk baby snoozing in your arms. You could sit there all day and just stare at him – and if you're not too tired, you should! Although, if you can bear to tear yourself away from him, once you're sure he's sleeping soundly pop him in his Moses basket and get forty winks yourself! Chances are you're just as tired, and you don't want to run the risk of nodding off with him on the sofa. You'll both sleep better separately, and getting him used to sleeping away from you, if only two feet away, is a good habit to get into from very early on, one that will stand you in good stead for that golden sleep routine later on.

> As long as your baby is full, he'll probably be asleep before he's even finished a feed.

I think that for the first month or so, do whatever is necessary to get your baby to sleep. Some solutions are more extreme than others – such as driving your baby around in the middle of the night until he falls asleep. But who am I to say this is wrong? I thought I had child-rearing nailed after Harry and Belle, but then Chester came along and, let me tell you, if I'd thought driving him around in the car for an hour a night would work, I'd have done it! Anything goes, and whatever works for you and keeps you sane in those early days is worth a punt.

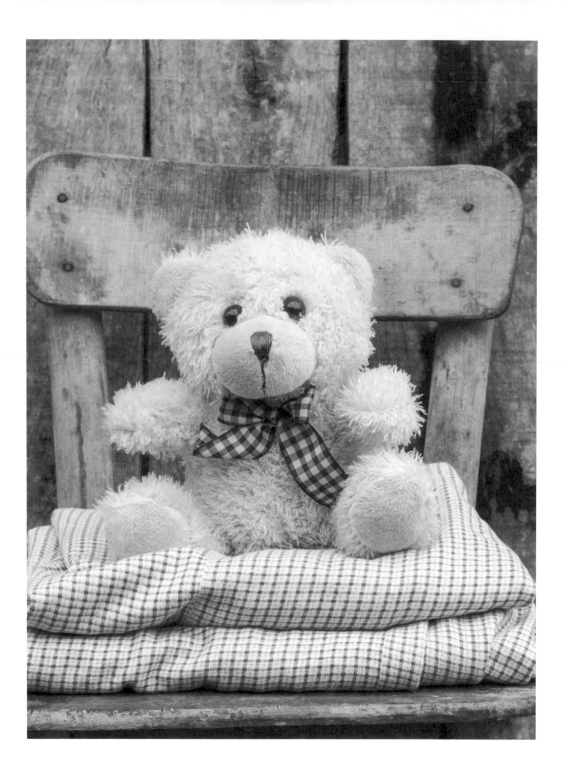

When your baby is about three months old you may want to start establishing a routine. Here are some helpful ways to kick things off:

Distinguish between day and night Whilst you're getting to grips with feeding and the continuous exhaustion you feel during the first few weeks, one thing you can do very easily to prepare your baby for getting into a good routine is to help him differentiate between day and night. It doesn't take any commitment from your baby, just an awareness from you that once 'night' falls, any time from about 7pm, you make every effort to keep the lights low, the noise down, the atmosphere calm and try not to interact too much with your baby when feeding. The ultimate goal is to get him to sleep for longer periods through the night than during the day, so that eventually he'll be sleeping for the whole night. If you don't encourage him to make this distinction, he may end up in a 24-hour cycle of eating and sleeping, with no idea that he's keeping you up all night when you should all be fast asleep!

Equally, during the daytime, don't tiptoe around too much if your baby is asleep. If it's your first baby, it's easy to be silent in the early days when he is sleeping – not so much if it's your second or third, with other children being manic around you! If you've ever visited other first-time mothers in the early days, you may have noticed an extraordinary feeling of peace that falls over a house where there's a sleeping newborn. The lights are dimmed and the house is warm and cosy – whilst this is all very lovely, it's better not to get a baby too used to that quiet. Your baby doesn't need complete silence – think back to how he slept in that noisy hospital after the birth – it's something you introduce into their lives, knowingly or not, so I would say keep the ambient sounds going whilst your baby's having a nap. There will come a point where you actually want to put the hoover on and if your baby hasn't learnt to block out noises you're going to have a problem. If you keep daytimes fairly busy and night-times peaceful, it won't be long before your baby sleeps for longer stretches at night than during the day, which is exactly the sleep pattern you want!

I'm a big advocate of not being too quiet around a sleeping baby – start as you mean to go on.

Regular daytime sleeps During the first few weeks you'll notice your baby becoming more and more aware of what's going on around him during the day. There will be times when he has his eyes wide open to a blurry world, trying to make sense of it and, as a result, might not be sleeping as much as he was. When he's asleep he may be disturbed more easily. I can't stress how important it is that your baby sleeps well during the day, as regular daytime napping paves the way for regular night-time napping! If you let him go too long without a sleep, he'll be so overtired you'll struggle to get him to sleep in the evening when it really counts.

As a rule of thumb for the first couple of months, most babies need to go back to sleep between one and two hours after being awake – this includes feeding time, so try to get your baby into a pattern very early on. Once he has a full tummy, has been winded and had a nappy change, and has been awake for an hour or so, try putting him down in the Moses basket or carrycot for a snooze. Sometimes he'll be so busy looking around he might not think he's ready for a sleep, but you know best – remember that!

I can't recall who it was that told me sleep breeds sleep, but they were absolutely right and it was one of the best pieces of advice I was given. Moreover, when you put a satisfied, changed baby down awake or semi-awake, you're also teaching him the most valuable skill of all when it comes to sleep training: how to settle himself to sleep. The earlier your baby learns to go to sleep without the help of anything or anyone, the better. Perfecting how to self-settle is literally the Holy Grail of sleep training. Once your baby nails that, you're on the home stretch when it comes to an undisturbed night's sleep. Even if something wakes him, he'll be able to get himself back to sleep. Having had three babies, all of whom I put down awake as much as I could, I've ended up with three excellent sleepers, and am not at risk of spending the next 10 years lying on the floor next to their beds until they fall asleep!

Recognise the sleepy signs In order to help your baby get into a good sleep routine you need to learn his sleepy signals so that you don't miss a single daytime napping opportunity. As well as doing all the usual things, such as yawning and rubbing his eyes, your baby might get red, heavy eyes or cry uncontrollably before falling asleep in the same breath as he was previously screaming. Belle used to pull her ears when she was tired, and I knew it was time for bed.

Even if your baby only naps for half an hour, make the most of that sleepy window – he might get a second wind, which is the last thing either of you want. If your baby misses a much-needed nap, he will soon become over-tired and too over-emotional to sleep without considerable help later in the day. It's no different to when you're shattered from a manic day at work and desperate to sleep, but when your head hits the pillow your mind won't shut down enough to let you. Awake time is so exciting for your baby – seeing your face, making sense of his surroundings – it's only natural that the more he wakes up to the world, the less he wants to close his eyes to it. So the onus is on you to spot when he's tired and save him from himself.

Another point worth mentioning here is that if your baby falls asleep in the daytime only to be disturbed and wake up again after a short time, don't be too quick to pick him up. He wants to sleep, you know that, so first try just letting him know that you are there by stroking him or shhhing him and see if he goes back off. If he doesn't, by all means try something else to settle him. The idea isn't for both of you to get in a state just to get your baby to sleep, but it's worth trying to see just how much comforting he needs before you pick him up and disturb him fully. Babies get tired very quickly from stimulation, and that can be as simple as looking at your face. Everything's so new to them that just taking it all in becomes exhausting.

Floppy arm To check whether your baby is in a deep sleep and ready to be placed in his cot, pick up his arm, and if it drops down heavily, he's ready. If it's still a bit stiff, wait a bit longer.

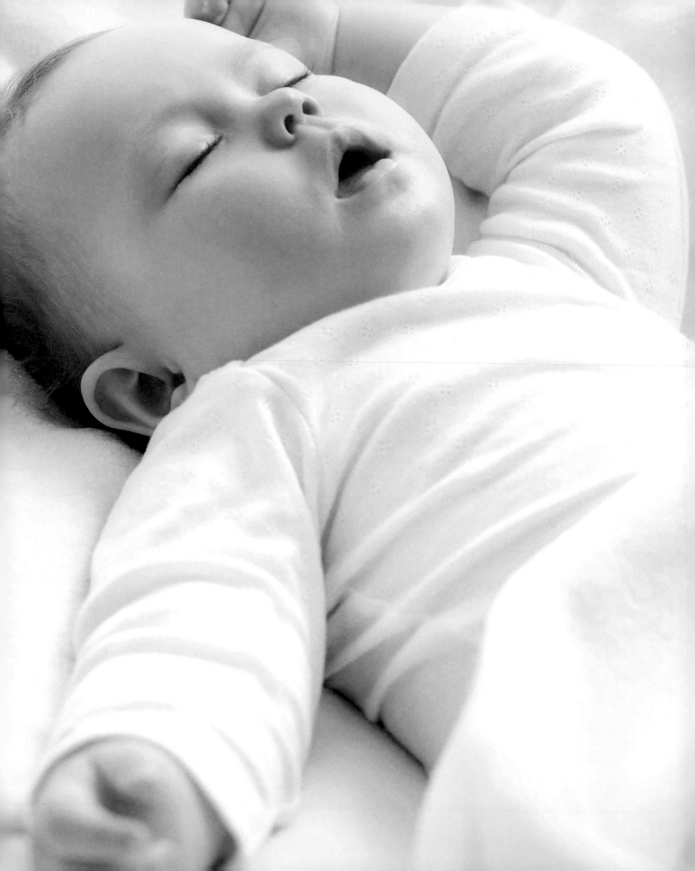

On the following pages I've shared the routines I used for all of my babies. See what you think, and then adapt them to suit you and your baby.

I expect you'll wonder how on earth you're going to keep on top of all these timings, and it's normal to feel that way. Whether you're reading this before your baby has arrived, or whether he's here already, such routines probably sound too straightforward and idealistic to ever work in practice – and you're not entirely wrong. Babies never do anything by the book and some days the routine will slip beyond belief, but if you can try to pull it back by the end of the day, at least you'll all get a good night's sleep, regardless of what's gone wrong during the day. Tomorrow is another day, so just have another go at getting it right then.

A few general things apply across all these routines:

First, a hungry baby is not going to go to sleep. A full baby will sleep before he's even finished a feed, but don't let that happen too early on. You'll need to encourage your baby to wake if he's nodding off after two minutes, but if it's been half an hour and his arms are dropping to his side like a lead weight, wind him, change him, wrap him up and put him down. The burping might even wake him up enough to finish his feed, which is your best-case scenario as a full tummy is what you're aiming for.

Second, bear in mind that a baby's sleep cycle is about 40 minutes. So whenever your baby has a nap, in an ideal world, it will be for a minimum of 40 minutes or he won't feel the full benefit. It's a bit like completing a full feed and not snacking before the next one. Your baby needs to complete a full sleep cycle and not 'snack' on sleep before it's time for the next nap, or you'll end up with lots of little ten-minute naps, which are of no use to anyone.

Third, you'll soon learn that your baby will go through phases. These can last anything from two weeks to two months! Some are worse than others, but frustratingly they all invariably mess with your routine! A lot of parents are initially blessed with 'model' babies, who sleep well from birth, only to find from three weeks it all goes out of the window when they decide to throw an hour of their own into the mix – the witching hour – usually daily at about 5pm!

All of mine hit this fussy phase at around five or six weeks, and they wouldn't settle in the evening until late. One of the reasons for prolonged crying at this time of day might be colic (see page 75), but apparently these fussy stages are often linked to their mental and physical development – once they pass, you might notice they've suddenly got taller, or they've learnt a new trick or two. They all go through it and, annoyingly for you, the fussiness always seems to come at the end of the day when you're absolutely exhausted and just want to put your feet up. It's particularly unfair that the witching-hour phase often starts at a time when your partner has gone back to work and any other help you might have been offered has evaporated! You could express off a feed or make up a bottle for your partner to give once he gets home, so you can get your head down between 8pm and the first night feed. I'm sure he'll be only too happy to take over and have some quality time with the baby he's been missing like crazy all day long, and you get to catch up on some sleep.

The only other thing I can say is to cuddle your way through it. If your fussy baby is only calmed by mummy cuddles, then cuddle away. If he wants to suckle at the breast for hours, then do it. Sometimes, routine is secondary, and this is one of those times. You'll get it back in a few weeks.

Finally, don't follow these routines too rigidly. If your baby wakes up at 8am, then adjust your routine to start from then. It's all about the space between naps, rather than what time your baby goes down or wakes up. Don't start your day when your baby first wakes up if it's 5am, or you'll never make it through the day. Treat any time he wakes up before about 6am as night-time – feed him and put him back down to sleep, then your day can begin when he next wakes, hopefully at a more sociable hour. Equally, though, try not to start your day any later than about 8am or you'll be so behind your timings by the end of the day that your baby may not be tired enough for bed at 7pm.

THE NATURAL NEWBORN ROUTINE
(BEFORE 6 WEEKS)

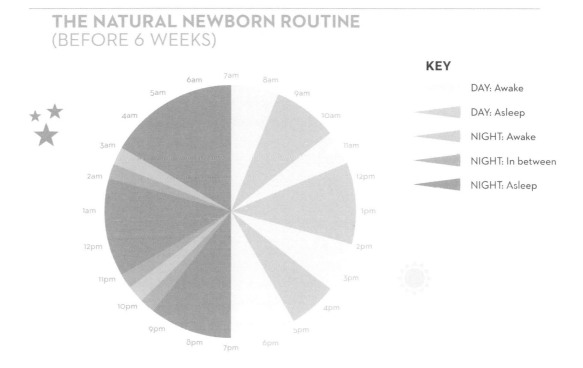

KEY

- DAY: Awake
- DAY: Asleep
- NIGHT: Awake
- NIGHT: In between
- NIGHT: Asleep

SLEEPING

Helpful hints Most newborns won't have any real pattern to how long and how often they sleep. You just have to know that they need it and let them have it, whether it's a catnap or a marathon sleep. However, and this might sound crazy, I'm giving you this super-early routine because you just might notice your baby falling into a natural sleeping pattern very early on, and I'm conscious about catering for every eventuality, no matter how unlikely!

THE PRE-ROUTINE
(6 WEEKS–3 MONTHS)

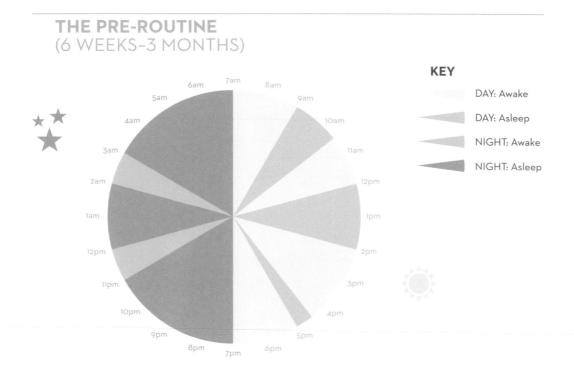

KEY

DAY: Awake

DAY: Asleep

NIGHT: Awake

NIGHT: Asleep

Helpful hints Three months is the time you really want to make sure your baby is settling into a routine. But you might notice one beginning to take shape the more food his tummy can hold, because he can nap for longer until the next feed. You'll also notice some of the sleep times are slightly later as he gets older. This is because he can stay awake for longer. You can help the routine by putting him down for a nap at certain times, as above. If your baby isn't waking up at the times you want him to, then adjust the time you put him down or give him a slightly longer morning nap. What you're working towards is the golden bedtime of 7pm (or whatever time suits your household), so the important thing is that he is tired enough to go down for the night at 7pm.

As all of mine neared three months old the routines shifted, whereby the morning sleep started happening a little later and was a little shorter. Like-wise, the afternoon nap becomes shorter. The biggest nap of the day becomes the lunchtime nap, which is why, where possible, I used to make sure I put them down in the cot in their rooms with the curtains closed for that nap, to try to maximise their chance of sleeping for a good chunk of time. But the other naps happened wherever we happened to be at the time. Babies need to fit in with your life as much as possible. You don't want to be fearful of stray-ing too far away from your baby's bedroom in case he needs a sleep!

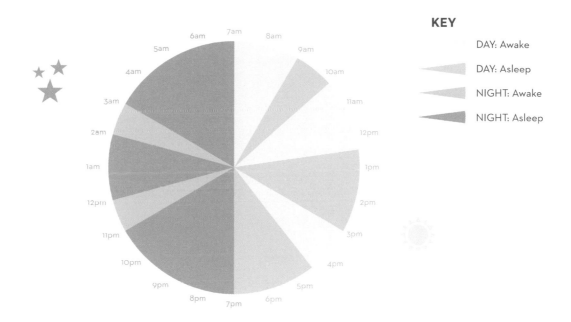

KEY

DAY: Awake

DAY: Asleep

NIGHT: Awake

NIGHT: Asleep

Helpful hints By three months it's helpful to develop a bedtime routine (see overleaf). A baby's body clock needs setting, consistency is key, and he will quickly respond to a set bedtime.

By about four months your baby should be able to handle a four-hourly feeding schedule, so try to eke him out to this if you can and fit your naps around it. Do of course amend the timings on my routine if your baby wakes earlier or later. It's the length of the gaps in between that are important. Try not to let your baby sleep for the last couple of hours before bedtime or he won't go down at that time. I tried not to let my babies sleep past 5pm.

At around five months your baby may no longer need an afternoon nap, so move the lunchtime one to around 1pm. If he's sleeping for a couple of hours then, he'll be more than happy to stay awake until bedtime at 7pm.

If your baby wakes in the night at this stage, it might not be because he is hungry. The first time he wakes you can try waiting to see if he'll be able to settle himself back to sleep without a feed.

SLEEPING

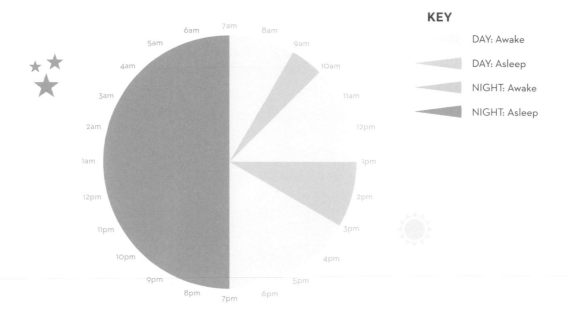

KEY

DAY: Awake

DAY: Asleep

NIGHT: Awake

NIGHT: Asleep

Helpful hints I found that Belle dropped her morning sleep at around twelve months and was quickly down to one nap a day, but Chester was slower to drop it, so be led by your child's particular needs. They're all different and burn up different amounts of energy at different times. As long as the amount of time your baby is asleep in the day in total stays the same, how it's broken up doesn't matter. If you find your little one reacts better to a long morning sleep and a shorter lunchtime sleep, then do it. Be guided by him. If you find he's not settling down to sleep at lunchtime, it could be because he doesn't need his morning sleep any more. All the routines are adaptable, and you'll know best how to tailor them to your baby's needs. If your baby is sleeping well through the night, whatever you're doing during the day is right. It's only when he stops sleeping well at night that you need to look at how his day sleeps might be impacting on this and adjust nap times slightly.

As your baby gets older it's a good idea to make sure both you and your partner are doing the bedtime routine, so that your baby doesn't become reliant on one parent. You'll make a rod for your own back if only you can put your baby down. By opening it up to a partner, it means that your baby will be far more receptive to others (grandma, friend, etc.), giving you the freedom to go out at night.

The big bedtime routine...

The sooner you can start a bedtime routine, the better – again, around three months is perfect. Your baby may not respond much in the early days, but I would say that once your baby stops seeing bath water as the enemy (see page 176), you can start. I've followed this bath and bedtime routine with all three of my babies, and whilst some things might change as your family grows and there are more children to throw in the bath of an evening, the basics remain the same!

A bath kicks off the evening bedtime routine, so you're looking to do it about half an hour before you actually want to put your baby down to sleep for the night. (This may start a bit earlier, depending on how many children you have to bath and dress for bed!)

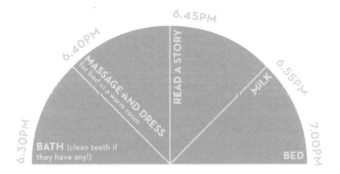

Once you run the bath, don't bring your baby back into the bustling day-time environment. If you're bottle-feeding, put everything you need in the baby's room. Keep things calm, with minimal stimulation. I would turn all the ceiling lights down or off and use lamps. It's all about getting the message across that it's time to sleep. If you dress your baby in the bathroom, let him have a naked kick around or do a bit of baby massage (see pages 186-7). For you, there is nothing more divine than the smell of a freshly bathed baby in a clean babygro and your baby gets the benefit of being warm, cosy and having you close.

I always read to Harry after his bath. It doesn't matter that young babies don't understand the words, it's your voice they love. When your baby is fed and winded, if he hasn't already nodded off into a milky stupor, put him down awake, say goodnight and close the door. Sounds simple, right?! Keep to the same routine each night and it will become just that.

It's worth remembering that about 30 minutes before a baby becomes sleepy, his melatonin (the body's natural sleep hormone) levels increase. This is triggered by a decrease in light, so as soon as you take your baby into a dimly lit room you have a 30-minute window to get him fed and down or you risk losing out on that lovely melatonin.

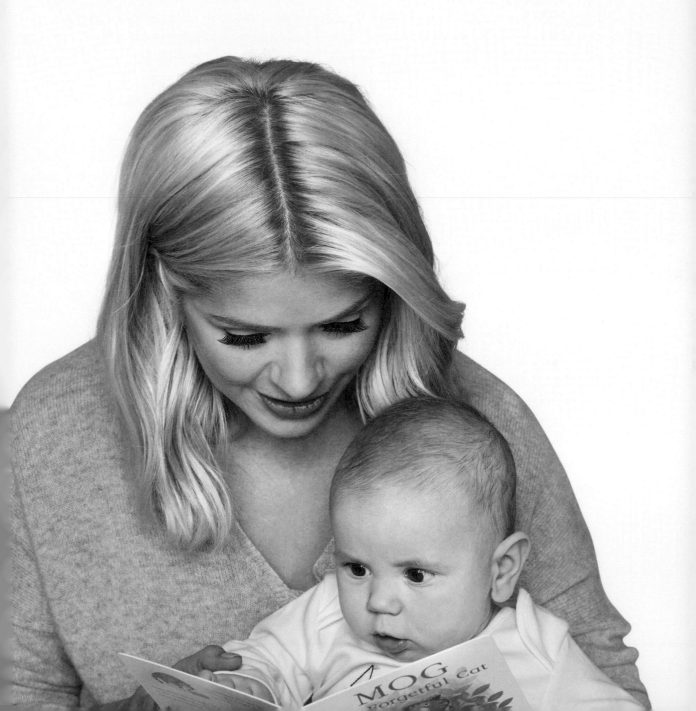

If your baby is poorly or teething and in pain, your sleep routine is likely to go out of the window. It's frustrating, because your baby will inevitably catch a dreadful cold or start sprouting really painful teeth precisely when you feel like you've cracked the sleeping thing and have had a really good run. Don't get despondent. Your baby won't forget everything he's learnt just like that, but you will have to be on hand for night care and cuddles when he is ill. The only thing you can try to stick to is the bath and bedtime routine and putting him down at the usual time, but the chances are your baby's appetite will have been affected so he may wake up hungry in the night. Do whatever you need to to get your baby through this rough patch. There's nothing more heartbreaking than a baby who looks so sorry for himself. Whatever the problem, hopefully these sleepless, poorly times will be few and far between.

Teething and cold remedies If your baby is teething, give him a dose of infant paracetamol for pain relief and he will hopefully settle back to sleep after about 15 minutes, once it's kicked in. In the meantime, he'll undoubtedly need a good cuddle! If your baby is streaming with a cold, you could try a baby cold medication, but be careful with some of the room and chest decongestants as you can't give them to a baby under three months old. There are some chest rubs you can use, which release a light eucalyptus vapour to help clear the sinuses. Before that, though, you're really at the mercy of saline drops and sprays to try to clear their nasal passages to help them sleep – or those contraptions you can suck the snot out with. It isn't as disgusting as it sounds and they do work, as I learnt with Chester! I think I was too nervous to try them with Harry or Belle!

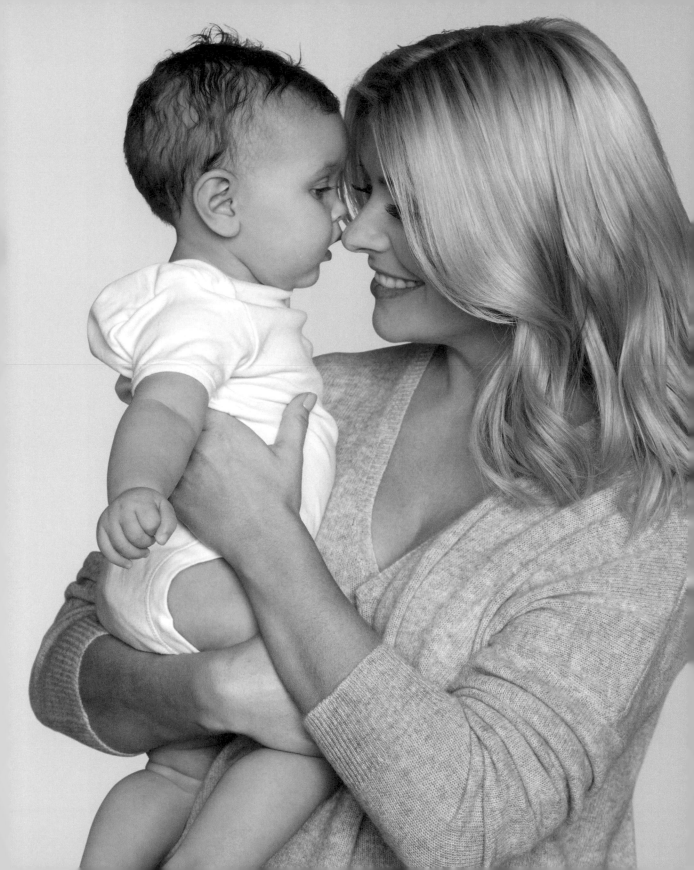

03 Sleep solutions

There are a million and one – probably more! – sleep solutions to help you and your baby achieve a perfect night's sleep, but be mindful that as soon as you start something with a baby, you create a habit. Just ensure that you do your research, and don't try anything you aren't happy to keep up for the next year or so!

My advice is to start small and hope that the little things help to settle your baby, like swaddling or patting his bottom rhythmically, before you move to the more dramatic solutions, such as driving around the M25 for the entire witching hour! When you're in a fraught, sleepless nightmare, it can make you feel desperate and, if that's you, just remember that nothing lasts forever and hopefully there will be something here for you to try that actually helps.

Remember, too, to keep trying things. As babies enter different phases, something that had no effect at all during fussy week four might be a cure at eight weeks. The key with all of these solutions isn't to knock your baby out cold, but to get him to a level of calm where you can put him down to settle himself to full sleep.

TROUBLESHOOT:
WHY WON'T MY BABY SLEEP?

There are so many things that can wreak havoc with your baby's sleep, so before you start throwing *your* toys out of the pram, go through this mental checklist for an explanation. Some you can remedy right away, some you might have to wait until tomorrow to do differently, and others might simply be a phase you have to patiently wait to pass.

Over-tired? **Has your baby not had enough daytime sleeps?**

Over-stimulated? **Babies respond better at bedtime if they've had a calm run-up.**

Dirty or wet nappy? **Does your baby need changing … again?!**

Ill? **Does your baby have a temperature or is he full of cold? If he's ill, routines fall apart.**

Teething? **If your baby is teething, give him a dose of infant paracetamol. After about 15 minutes he'll be ready to go back down again.**

Comforter? **Has he lost it somewhere in the cot and is crying because he can't find it?**

Dummy? **Is it constantly falling out and waking him up?**

Too much sleep? **Has he had too much sleep during the day or a late sleep too close to bedtime? Where possible, try to keep your baby awake for two hours before bedtime.**

Hungry? **Is he snacking all day, so not filling up at mealtimes?**

Too many night feeds? **Are you feeding him at night to get him to go back to sleep? If yes, he won't be as hungry in the daytime, so won't fill up as much at mealtimes. Try to regulate the day feeds so he has enough in his tummy before bed to make him sleep longer through the night.**

Growth spurt? **Is he going through a growth spurt or about to reach a milestone of some sort? This may make him ravenous, so bring back an extra feed for this phase.**

Rock and shhh technique ...

I think babies like being rocked or patted because it reminds them of being in the womb and moving about with you, which is also why they tend to nod off in the pram as soon as you start moving. Try not to get into a habit of doing anything too energetic as you rock your baby to sleep. If you start you'll have to keep it up. I always found rhythmic bottom-patting soothed all of mine and I used to tap out a heartbeat rhythm on their back whilst making shhhing and ahhhh sounds.

Swaddling ...

Swaddling must be the oldest way of comforting a baby to sleep. It's essentially a technique where you wrap your baby up so he's snug and contained. Whilst there's definitely a knack to doing it, once you've got it it can be very effective. The most important thing to remember is to make sure your baby's head isn't covered in any way and to make sure you use breathable materials, such as a large muslin or one of the special cellular baby blankets, as you don't want your baby to overheat – and never swaddle above the shoulders or swaddle him too tightly. Consider the conditions around you and decide on the appropriate clothing for your baby to wear under the swaddle cloth. You should also check your baby's temperature when swaddled to make sure he's not too hot.

Be guided by your baby as they're all different. Whilst some hate to feel restricted and will fight it, some like the sense of being completely confined, as if they're back in the womb. Belle was definitely one of those babies. I think because she was premature and so tiny, she really loved being swaddled – the tighter the better made her feel cuddled and secure. I swaddled Harry for a different reason. He used to startle himself awake. His arms would fly up in the air all of a sudden and he'd twitch, so a light swaddle helped to keep him asleep longer.

My niece on the other hand couldn't bear to have her arms and hands constricted and hated being swaddled, so my sister compromised on a sort of half-swaddle under the arms. That way she was warm and cosy, but not restricted and frustrated! Chester was similar to my niece in that he didn't seem to like having his hands constricted by his sides. As luck would have it, I found an all-in-one sleeping bag that zipped up the middle, incorporating his hands up by his head – which is the preferred way for most babies to sleep. Very clever!

Try a sling I used to walk around the house with Chester in a sling. This kept him upright whilst asleep, which was best for his reflux issues. The added bonuses of this are that it allows you to be hands-free to get on with chores and, as your baby grows and gets heavier, it saves your back!

Settling holds ...

There are so many different types of holds to try to make your baby feel calm and on the way to 'sleepy'. Here are some of the classic ones:

Settling your baby on your lap I learnt a great lap-settling trick for babies up to about three months old, from sleep expert and author Alison Scott-Wright, where you put a pillow on your lap and lay your baby on his tummy with his head turned to the side. Then you rhythmically pat your baby's back above his nappy until he drops off to sleep. I did this with Chester and found that even though he cried to begin with, after a few minutes he was sound asleep – and all that from the comfort of the sofa! Just remember that the safest position for babies to sleep is on their back (see pages 91–93), so don't leave your baby sleeping on his tummy if this trick works for you.

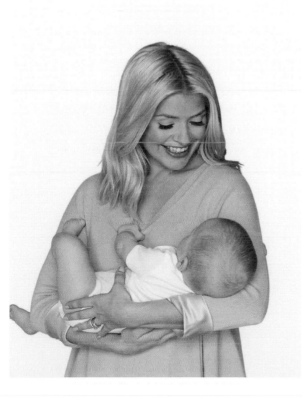

Cradle carry hold The cradle carry is the classic baby hold, where your baby's head rests in the bend of your cradled arms, whilst he gazes up at you, which is comforting for both you and him.

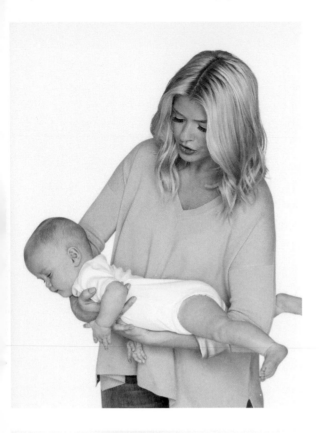

Rugby ball hold Babies seem to love this position where you lay them face down along your forearm, with their head and neck resting in the bend of your cradled arm for support. Apparently, the pressure on their tummy is good for helping to relieve any trapped wind and they have the freedom to look out at the world.

Swaying-seat hold (made that name up!) In this hold you use your body and hands to make a seat for your baby so that he can face out and look at the world. Use one hand under his bottom to make the seat base and support his back against your stomach. Then move around the room or just sway from side to side. Babies love this hold, but it can wreak havoc with your back as they get heavier. Once they reach the age they can face out in a baby carrier, it's essentially the same hold but with straps rather than hands.

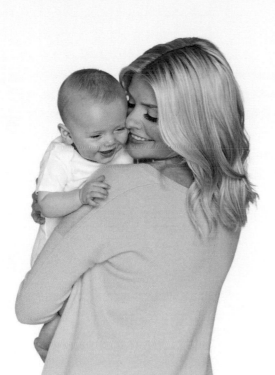

Over-the-shoulder hold This is also a good position to give your baby a different view. Lay him upright against your shoulder, with his head peeking over the top (support his head with your hand if he needs it). This is the ideal position to tap him on the back and release any trapped wind. I'd recommend placing a muslin over your shoulder, though, or you might end up with some vomit down your back!

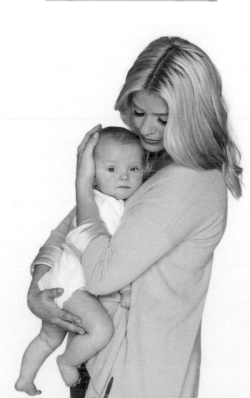

Heartbeat hold Hold your baby to your chest facing in, supporting his bottom, back and neck, with his head resting near your heartbeat. This is the sound he's most familiar with and will find most comforting. You can wrap him up in a sling like this to save your arms too.

Slowly lowering into the cot ...

Quite often, if my babies fell asleep on me when I was holding them after a feed, they would wake up the moment I put them in the cot. As soon as I moved them away from me, where they'd been warm and snuggly, and the cold air rushed into the gap between us, they'd wake straight up. I found that if I started moving them away really slowly, inch by inch, until they were lying flat out in front of me on my arms, there was no sudden drop in temperature, and very slowly I could put them down in their cot. Try it – it worked for me!

Touching and cuddling ...

Cuddles are the best! Keeping your baby close and stroking him gently and rhythmically can send him off into a deep sleep. And it's good for you to get all that yummy oxytocin flowing. As well as cuddles, a little bit of baby massage (see pages 186–7) can be a magical part of a baby's bedtime routine. This can be as simple as rubbing oil or baby lotion into your baby's body. Think what would feel nice to you and do the same for your baby, very lightly. If you're worried about being too heavy handed, just use your two middle fingers to make light, circular motions. I did this with all of mine, especially after a bath, laying them on a towel on the floor in the warm bathroom.

I couldn't lay Chester down flat because of the reflux, but I knew he would really benefit from a calming massage before bed. I ended up raising the top of his changing mat to a 45-degree angle, laying him on his tummy and then putting a baby mirror in front of his face, which stopped him from wriggling whilst I massaged. Apparently his own face was the most fascinating thing in the world!

Use your voice ...

Your voice, combined with your touch, is the single most calming thing your baby can experience. Speak to your baby in soothing tones or sing. Repeated songs and tunes soon become familiar to your baby and a real comfort.

SOLUTIONS: EXTRA THINGS TO TRY

White noise ...

Having had three children, my house is never quiet, so Chester didn't have any choice but to sleep through noise. That child would sleep through an earthquake! I have to say, though, I did buy one thing that I think really helped him block out external noises and drift off to sleep, and that was a white noise machine. I got it for him because I didn't think it was fair to leave the onus on him of blocking out two noisy children tearing around the house.

It's a little machine you plug in next to the cot that mimics the white noise sound you get in between radio stations. You can also get white noise apps for when you're out and about, and even everyday things at home might have the same effect. I can remember my sister saying that my niece Lola went through a phase of dropping off as soon as she started drying her hair. So sometimes, if she was having difficulty getting her to sleep, she'd run the hairdryer for a minute or so in the background and it would do the trick! (Obviously don't leave a running hairdryer unattended!)

There is some research that found that listening to white noise helps all of us, not just children, go into a deeper sleep, and that the quality of sleep you get is better and you are more refreshed after a two-hour sleep with white noise than without it. External sounds disturb you whilst you sleep, whether you remember when you wake or not. By sleeping with one continuous sound, there's not such a jump between silence and one of those external noises, so you're less likely to be disturbed and therefore sleep better.

Night-lights and soothing music ...

Be careful not to make a rod for your own back with night-lights or soothing music. I think a baby that learns to settle himself is the baby you want in your life. A night-light is something you buy for your child, probably because you think he needs it, or it looks pretty in the nursery. Remember that whatever you start with becomes normal for your baby. Why introduce something in those early days, when your baby actually has no idea what's going on? Months later, when you've decided to have a weekend away at a lovely hotel for some quality family time, you'll get to bedtime to discover you've forgotten your child's changing-colour star-projector light and music box and all hell will break loose! Are you prepared to risk that weekend becoming memorable for all the wrong reasons?! Also the majority of baby night-lights have blue lights in them somewhere, which is really stimulating before bedtime. For the same reason, you shouldn't have your mobile phone shining blue by your bed. If you are going to go down the night-light route, choose a warm colour, something red or yellow.

You want to be able to put your baby down in his cot with his eyes open and say, 'Night, night,' and walk out of the room, leaving him to drift off to sleep on his own. And babies do! They really do! I think there's so much temptation to rock a baby to sleep and then put him down, but bear in mind that whatever you start you're stuck with, unless you go through the misery of cold turkey trying to break a habit further down the line. That will be no fun for either of you (even though I swear you can break any habit within three days!) – so it's just best not to start.

Comforters …

A comforter, in whatever form you choose, be it a soft toy or a blankie, can help your baby feel secure if he wakes during the night and you're not there. The guidelines tell you not to put anything in the cot with your baby before six months (see page 86–7), but after that it might be worth introducing one.

Cuddly toy rabbits were a real comfort for all of my babies – once they got to a certain age they would nuzzle the fur. As I used to snuggle with them, the toy had my scent on it, which meant they could smell me even though I wasn't there with them. It was just something that made them feel secure after I'd put them down to sleep in their cot, and, unlike a dummy, wasn't something they kept losing during the night.

Buy two! Make sure the comfort toy can be replaced if it's lost! In practice that's easier said than done, but we managed to lose Harry's at an airport in Scotland one weekend and I spent the day after we arrived home trying to track it down – which amazingly I did! After that disaster, I tried running two rabbits alongside each other with Harry, so he'd always have one if the other had to go in the washing machine. But, and don't ask me how, he always knew when he didn't have his original rabbit. Crazy! See what I mean about making a rod for your own back?!

Dummies ...

All three of my children have had dummies, and all three of them had them taken away at three months. For me a dummy was purely a tool to get them over those first few months of life – in particular, when they were crying excessively and needed calming to go to sleep – but it's up to you whether you use one and, if you do, when you take it away. I decided to get rid of the dummies as soon as they started falling out when the children were asleep. This would wake them up, effectively having the reverse effect. At three months babies are young enough not to miss a dummy and it usually only takes a couple of days to break the cycle.

> If you don't leave it too long before getting the dummy fairy to take it away, a dummy can be very useful.

Dummies can be quite a discussion piece amongst new mothers. There are valid arguments for and against using one, but I feel if you use it as a tool for a short period and don't let it become a crutch, ending up with a toddler with a serious dummy habit, it's fine. On the positive side, dummies are said to help reduce the risk of cot death; they quickly soothe a fraught baby as the sucking calms them; they're better than sucking on fingers or thumbs – at least you can take a dummy away to protect teeth development. And, on the negative side, there's a school of thought that if you are breastfeeding and use a dummy in the early days, you can confuse a baby's latching technique (by the way, all of mine were breastfed and all had dummies – no confusion there!); long-term use of them leads to bucked teeth; dummies can be a bit like chewing gum for an adult and suppress appetite; and, lastly, if your baby permanently has a dummy in his mouth, he won't be inclined to practise talking and explore making sounds, which are so crucial to learning to speak. However, I've never met a person who couldn't speak because they had a dummy. Have you?!

Obviously hygiene is paramount. You should buy plenty of dummies and sterilise them as you would your baby's bottles, and if there are any splits in the rubber, throw them away as these can collect harmful bacteria.

Sleep-inducing foods ...

Some foods promote good sleep, so give these a go with your little one if they're at the weaning stage. Foods such as turkey and most poultry (ever wondered why you're all snoring on the sofa on Christmas Day!), bananas, avocados, eggs and oats contain tryptophan, a sleep-inducing chemical.

Get you and your baby some fresh air ...

If your baby won't stop crying and none of the usual settling tricks are working, there's no substitute for getting out of the house – for the benefit of both of you! Don't stay at home pacing up and down or you'll both end up getting more annoyed. Wrap yourselves up, come rain or shine, and go for a walk. The fresh air will help you to clear your head and might knock the baby out too!

If you haven't left the house for days, you may feel like a prisoner in your own home and need a change of scenery. Even if it's raining, put the rain-cover on the pram, grab yourself an umbrella or a waterproof with a hood and walk out. And I don't mean go and meet someone for a coffee, I mean just walk. You need clear head space. If you meet someone, it'll all become about the baby again. So, like I said, just get up and go for a short walk.

Now, I've been there on many occasions with all of mine: you step outside with a screaming baby and feel that he has the loudest cry in the world. You feel as if everyone's looking at you and wondering why you're not doing something to stop it. But actually the majority of people you walk past have either had or cared for children and they'll all recall going through a time just like that.

My mum swears by fresh air for babies. She used to wrap me up warm and wheel me out into the back garden for a snooze (under supervision, of course!), even if there was a frost on the ground. As long as we were snug and warm, and there wasn't a hurricane forecast, my sister and I spent a lot of our early life asleep out on the patio!

I've seen research that says babies sleep better at night after being exposed to daylight. The daylight suppresses the levels of melatonin in our system, then when it's dark the melatonin is released and gets your baby into a more natural pattern of sleeping. Anything that helps, eh?!

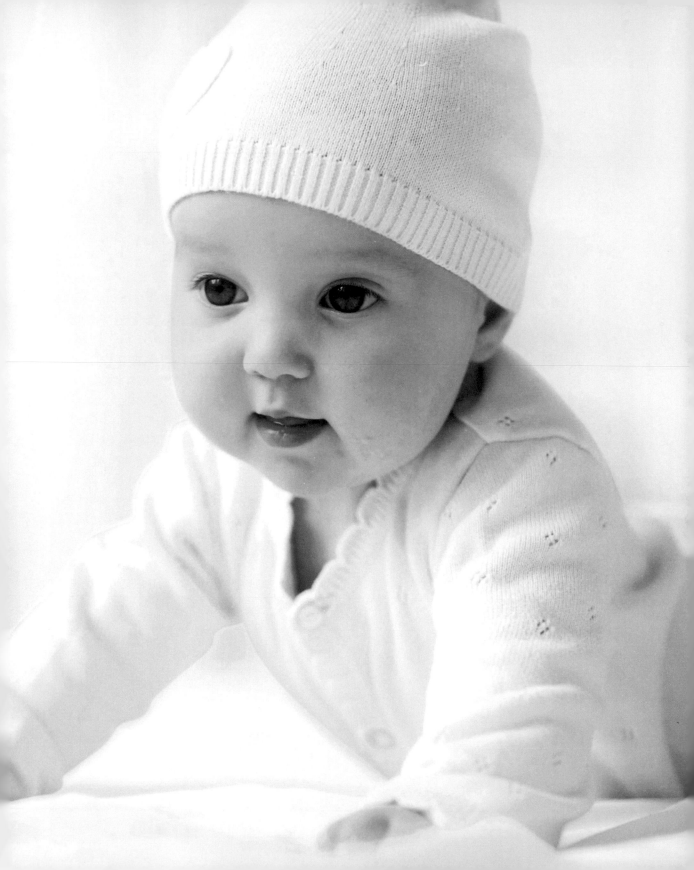

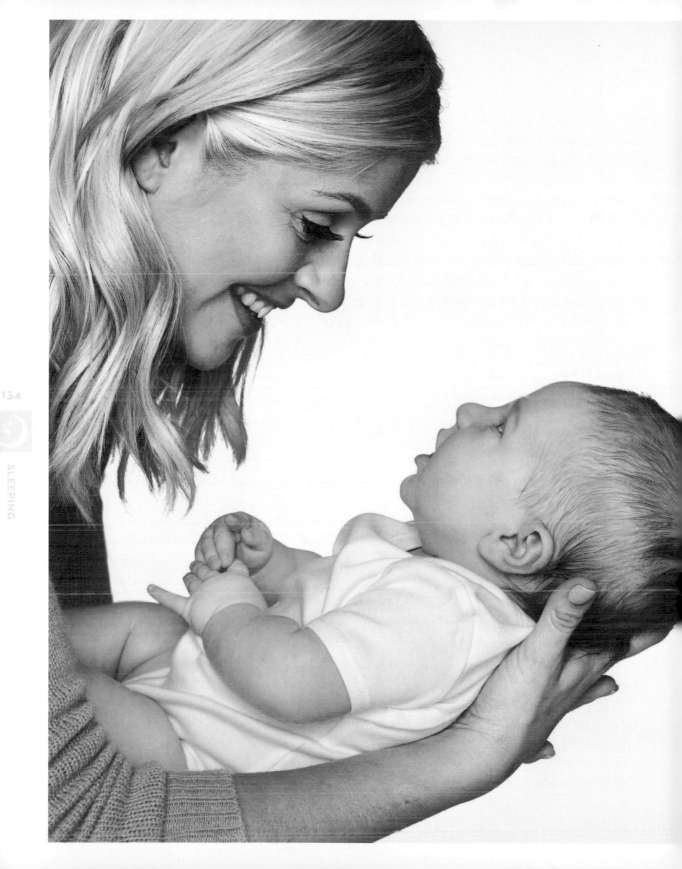

What worked for me ...

All three of mine were totally different and I adjusted things according to each baby's temperament and situation. If Chester cried out in the night, for example, I'd know he was in some sort of reflux pain and there was no way I was going to leave him. But by the time Harry was about four months old, if he cried out I knew he was fine – he was just having a bit of a whinge. I found that if I did go to him I'd end up making it so much worse. With both Harry and Belle, half the time I found that if I left them for a few minutes, even if I just stood outside the door and listened, more often than not they would settle themselves and go back to sleep, to the point where they got really good at it and stopped crying out at all if they were disturbed.

Judge the cry ...

Listen to what that cry is. There are different levels of crying, from a whinge to a hysterical, continuous cry. No mother wants to leave their baby crying, so it's important to emphasise that you're not here to harm, hurt or distress your baby in any way. However, if your baby is eight months old and is still waking up several times a night and you're running in every time, you and your baby are going to spend the following day utterly exhausted. If you're in that sleepless cycle, isn't it worth a few nights just seeing where those cries might lead to?

If you racing to answer every cry isn't making any difference as an hour later he's at it again, your baby is clearly not happy either. Bear in mind he might not even really be awake when he cries out, or he might have just bumped the side of the cot in his sleep and be reacting to that. If you go bowling in and pick him up before giving him a minute to go back off to sleep, you risk disturbing him fully, at which point he'll go really bananas! He was only twitching and he's now really annoyed not to be asleep any more, which means you have hit your worst-case scenario: it's the middle of the night, you have a grumpy baby, a broken routine and an even grumpier, tired mummy! It's likely that his night awakenings have just become a habit, a sleep pattern that needs breaking. It's worth learning how to help your baby to settle himself without your intervention. He isn't going to learn how to do that if every time he cries you run in – in a way you are doing more harm than good. But you know best! Listen to your gut feeling whether you need to go in or not.

Controlled crying ...

This technique teaches babies to fall asleep by themselves. The idea is that by leaving your baby to cry for increasing lengths of time before going in to comfort him, he will get better at settling himself and learn how to fall asleep on his own. I would definitely say don't consider controlled crying until your baby is six months old. Before that time, I think that if your baby is crying, he needs you. But, again, it really depends on the baby. All babies are different, and no one knows your baby better than you do, so listen to your motherly instinct to know what stage your baby is at; only you know your child enough to know if he's ready.

Sleep training ...

It's not easy to be strong when you hear your little one crying, and it will be exhausting, but if you can stick it out for three nights you won't believe the results. Here's how to do it: feed, wind and change your baby ready for

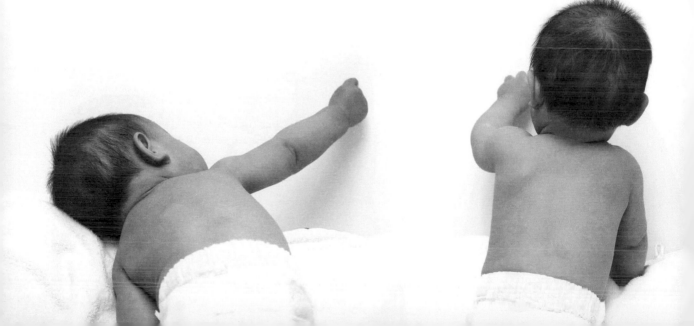

the 7pm bedtime, put him down in the cot awake or sleepy, give him a kiss and whisper, 'Night, night,' then walk out and gently close the door. Either he will be sleepy enough not to notice and drop straight off, or he'll start screaming. Listen and wait for any crying to stop. I would say leave it about ten minutes if the cries are slowing, and then – just when you think you should go in – wait another minute. So many times I've resisted going in and 30 seconds later there's a silent, sleeping baby. If the crying continues and your baby is getting himself into a state, then of course go in, but don't pick him up straight away. Reassure him you're there, give him his comforter if he's lost it and try to soothe him. If that doesn't work, move on to solutions, such as rocking him. Only offer a feed as a last resort. After three days of being strong, the initial ten minutes will drop to seven, then three, then he might only grizzle for a minute.

No one wants to hear a baby in distress, but I promise you that when the time is right (usually at some point after six months) within two or three days you could have a different child on your hands, one who is sleeping through the night. Consistency is the key. The only way to break a habit is to offer up a different one. Good luck!

I could pretend I had the answer to this but I'd be lying. I think I've been tired since I had Harry! But on the plus side, that crazy tiredness at the beginning, when it feels as if your baby is feeding every two minutes, does come to an end. You will be tired, but it won't be anything like those first couple of months.

Call on your partner …

In the first couple of weeks after your baby arrived, your partner probably couldn't have been more helpful. But you might find that starts to wane a little once he goes back to work and realises how difficult it is to function effectively on limited sleep. Work out a way for you to share the load, rather than both of you being present and awake night after night. Once he comes home from work (if it's not too late), let him help with the bath and bedtime routine. If you do everything yourself, your baby will only ever want mummy to do everything, so this is important to help him learn to be flexible. Then once you've done the first night feed, make sure there's an expressed or formula bottle ready for the second night feed for your partner to give, and go to bed! You might be able to get four hours sleep before you need to express off a feed, or even longer if you're formula feeding.

I think sometimes there's too much onus on the mum to get up every time a baby cries. I know you'll feel like ships in the night, but it's only for the first few months. What's most important is that you're both getting a decent amount of sleep every night and your partner is getting some much-needed one-on-one bonding time with the baby he misses all day long.

Dan and I have always shared the night-time parenting where possible. Yes, your partner may go out to work during the day, but your days are long and tough too – perhaps tougher! The times I've heard men say they'd rather be out at work, when they think their wife isn't listening! And, anyway, if you go on to have more than one child, you'll end up with one each to deal with during the night, so the quicker you both get used to working as a team, the easier it will all be and the more balanced and flexible your child will be.

Phone a friend …

The most reassuring thing I can tell you is that nothing ever lasts for that long – it's something I tell myself all the time! If your baby is going through a terrible sleeping phase, for example, after sleeping through the night for months, remember that it is just that, a phase, and it will come to an end. Nothing is forever. Thinking that way always helped me through the tougher days and nights with all of mine.

But don't be afraid to ask for help if you're really in a black hole! If you haven't slept for days and you're starting to feel you can't cope or go on, PHONE SOMEONE! Phone your mum or your mother-in-law, or your sister or your best mate! This is what these unwanted guests are for! Brilliant! 'You're here! Chester's just been fed. Would you mind taking him around the block? I just need to get my head down for an hour as I've been up all week!' Do you think they'll mind? Of course not. They'll know from the bags under your eyes that you'll love them forever for helping you in your time of need, and wouldn't ask unless you were absolutely desperate. And, anyway, let's not ignore the fact they might actually enjoy getting this gorgeous bundle of loveliness all to themselves, without you fussing over them.

Another thing I found to be an enormous comfort was other mums. This may sound weird, but I remember in the dead of night during those early months tweeting 'Morning fellow mummies' at some ridiculous hour and feeling so happy to receive a load of tweets from other exhausted feeding mummies! Just remember, you are not alone. There are always other mummies out there, and there are some brilliant online forums that you can join for a chat, a moan or some advice.

Summary Hopefully you've found a few things here that resonate with you and make sense. How best to get your baby to sleep is such an enormous discussion, and something everyone has an opinion on.

I've shared some of the key things that worked for me to help you troubleshoot your own situation, but listen to your instincts and trust your decisions. Try not to get down-hearted if you're struggling to get more than an hour's sleep at a time, which is, I know, easier said than done.

Communication with your support network is key to make sure you're getting enough help to allow you to catch up on your sleep when things are tough. And, remember, nothing lasts forever! All babies sleep through the night eventually.

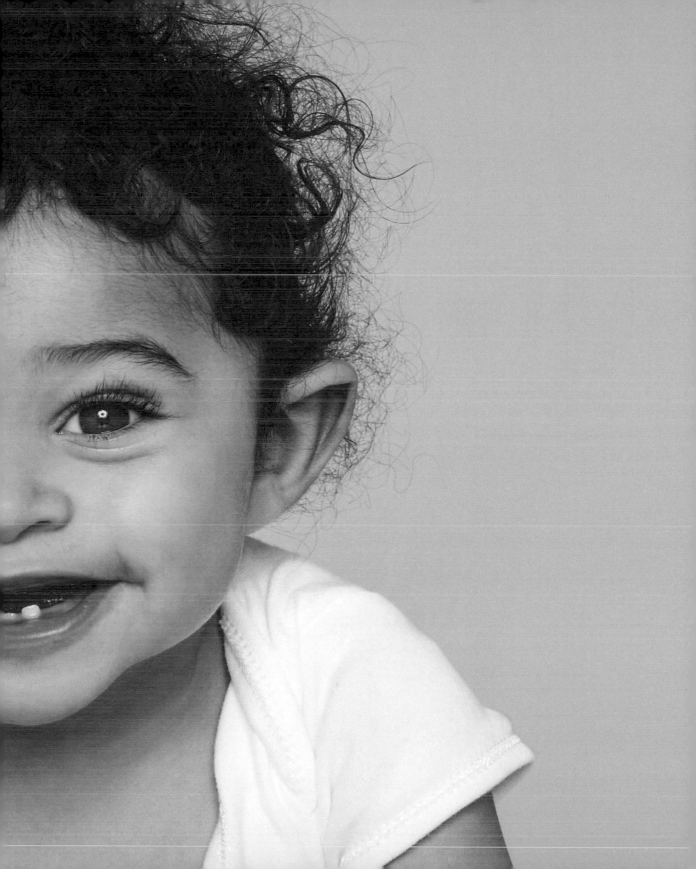

Wellbeing

- CHAPTER THREE -

+

My new baby is here. Now what do I do?!

First, don't panic! It's normal to doubt you can care for your newborn baby, but you most certainly can! You will grow in confidence every day, and caring for your little one will soon become second nature.

There's so much to think about and be aware of in your first year as a mum, and forewarned is most definitely forearmed. So in this chapter I want to give you a heads up about some of the things to expect and hopefully enlighten you a little – apologies in advance if there's a touch of TMI (too much information)! But believe me, when you go to change a nappy and discover the contents look like tar, you'll be glad I mentioned it! It's not all about bodily functions, however. I've covered things like how to bath your baby, the dos and don'ts of nappy changing, how to soothe your baby, how to cope with teething pain, what vaccinations she'll have and when to call the doctor. I've tried to share all the things I needed to know after having Harry, so hopefully you'll find some of the answers you're looking for here.

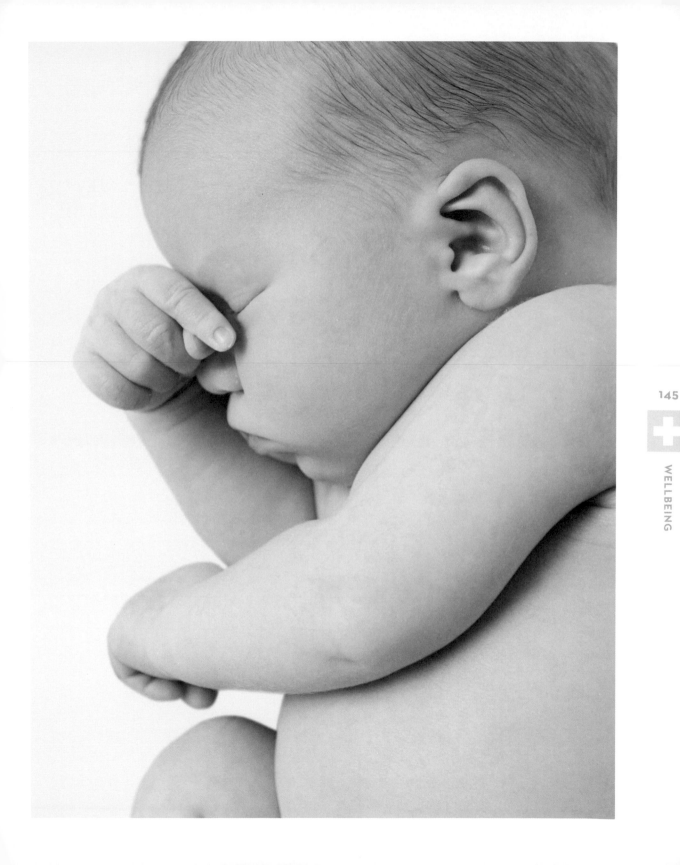

01 Your newborn's wellbeing

We all have a picture of our babies in our minds before they're born, but don't be shocked if your baby doesn't look anything like the ones in the movies!

Harry, was … eek … a forceps delivery, so on his perfect little face there were two long red welts, which stayed there for a few days. Belle arrived a bit jaundiced but after a few days of leaving her to sleep in her Moses basket in a room with lots of natural daylight (but not in direct sunlight!) all that lovely Vitamin D turned her a perfect shade of baby pink!

So in this section I've tried to give you some idea of what your newborn will look like so you know what to expect. I've also covered the harmless routine tests and checks your baby can expect immediately after birth and within the first week of her life, which ensures she is healthy and everything is in good working order.

HOW YOUR NEWBORN MIGHT LOOK

Most newborns have a slightly strange appearance, and there are numerous reasons for this. The majority of babies (of whatever ethnicity) are born a ruddy sort of purple, but they can vary in colour – anything from white to yellow, and, depending on how they've been lying in the womb all this time, their arms and legs might come out and want to remain at a slightly odd angle. A premature baby might still have some of the things that have usually disappeared by the time a baby reaches full term (such as a layer of soft downy hair; see below), and if you've had a difficult delivery some of the instruments and techniques used may have left their mark.

Another good example of an unusual arrival was my niece, Lola. Because she was breech for the last six weeks, she was delivered by planned Caesarean section, with two legs that wanted to remain up by her ears, and a head the shape of a rugby ball, which you can imagine was quite distressing for my sister at first. I can only assure you that Mother Nature is a miracle worker and within a couple of days everything from skin colour to misbehaving limbs ended up the way they should and little Lola is perfect!

My newborn is white: vernix During the last trimester your baby's skin is covered all over by a cheesy, white, greasy substance known as vernix, which has several jobs to do. It protected your baby's skin in the womb (think how wrinkly your skin gets when you've been in the bath too long!) and it's a very slippery substance, so it acts as a lubricant during the delivery. Not only does it help you push your baby out, it also keeps your baby's skin moisturised once she's out and provides an extra layer of warmth after the birth.

My newborn is hairy: lanugo Before babies are covered in vernix their hair follicles suddenly start working and their bodies develop a covering of downy, soft hair. Most babies lose this hairy layer in the womb, but occasionally it's still present after they're born, which can be slightly surprising! This is more common in premature babies (but not always!) who haven't completed their time in utero but, as with vernix, it's a good thing as it's another layer to keep them warm when they're first born.

My newborn is blue: too cold Your baby's hands and feet may look a bit blue if they get cold. Just keep an eye on them. They should turn pink again once they're warm. When your newborn cries excessively her lips may turn blue, but again that should disappear as soon as she calms down. If, however, your baby retains a permanent blue colour it might indicate a heart or lung problem, so seek medical help right away – particularly if you notice your baby is struggling to breathe.

My newborn is yellow: jaundice It's common for newborns to suffer from neonatal jaundice, which you'll know all about if your baby has a yellow tinge to her skin and the whites of her eyes. It's one of the first things your midwife will check for. Babies have more red blood cells in utero than they need in the outside world, so as soon as they are born they try to break these excess red blood cells down, creating a yellow substance called bilirubin. But because their livers are so tiny, it may take a while for them to get rid of all that bilirubin, which is what gives a baby a yellow hue! Your baby should return to a more normal pink colour within a week or so.

As I mentioned, getting Vitamin D through plenty of exposure to daylight can really help with this. If your baby is still yellow after a fortnight, or the jaundice doesn't actually begin to show until a week after birth, then seek medical help. It can be indicative of a more serious condition.

My newborn is bruised and swollen: forceps or ventouse delivery If you had a forceps delivery, it's likely your baby came out with a few scrapes or bruises, or some swelling where the forceps gripped her head. Likewise, a ventouse delivery will leave a small swelling on the head where the suction cup was attached. This all sounds awful, but don't feel mortified. The important thing is that your baby is safe and well and these marks will be gone before the week's out. You could also look into cranial osteopathy for your baby, which helps to relieve tension from these sorts of deliveries (see page 164).

My newborn is spotty: newborn rashes or spots Discovering skin imperfections on your baby can be quite distressing, but in nearly all cases any rashes or spots don't last for long and aren't painful. Most newborn rashes are a result of the mummy hormones your baby was exposed to during pregnancy.

Some newborns are born with a pink rash called neonatal acne and some with salmon patches, sometimes known as stork marks, which are little clusters of blood vessels usually on the back of the neck. Erythema toxicum is another common red blotchy rash, seen in around 50 per cent of newborns, and many also have milia, which are tiny little white spots, usually on the face. Of all the early skin conditions your baby might experience, it's only the salmon patches that might remain (possibly up to four years of age). Everything else is temporary. Definitely don't start squeezing any spots. Just continue to wash your baby as usual and these rashes and spots will naturally disappear.

Birthmarks We're all born unique, so you might find an unexpected birthmark somewhere on your newborn. Take me for example – I was born with a huge chocolate brown smudge across my right eyebrow, which my mum openly says she felt terrible about when I arrived. It was such a prominent mark on the tiny face of a newborn baby, and whilst it got smaller as I got bigger there are so many stories of me going 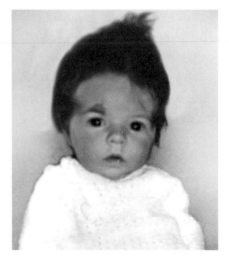 to friends' houses after school and their mothers scrubbing my face raw, to avoid sending me home with mud or chocolate on my face! But if you're feeling bad about it, don't! It's all these little things that make your child who they are. Your baby is perfect just the way they are.

NEWBORN TESTS AND PROCEDURES

Within the first minute of life ...

Cutting the umbilical cord The umbilical cord has literally been your baby's lifeline in the womb, and now your baby is here it's time for her to start doing things for herself. Quite often, Dad will have been asked whether he would like to cut the baby's cord after delivery, which he may or may not be up for doing! The cord is clamped in two places and cut, leaving a 2–3cm/1in stump that eventually turns black and drops off within a couple of weeks – what's then left is a tummy button!

Once you're home with your baby try to keep the area clean (see page 179) until the stump falls off. I can remember with all of mine, changing a nappy and discovering the cord had dropped off into it at some point. And then you'll be faced with the decision I think every parent goes through at that moment: 'What do I do with it? Do I keep it? Does it go in the baby memory box to be brought out at her 21st birthday?!' You might feel quite attached to it after all this time ('scuse the pun!). It's up to you, but don't say I didn't warn you when these weird thoughts come into your head!

Cord blood and stem cell transplants The blood within your baby's umbilical cord can be used later in life to treat many life-threatening conditions and there are companies that you can pay to freeze and store the whole cord. Then, should the worst happen and your child falls ill later in life, stem cells that are obviously a 100 per cent match to your child can be harvested to help. This is really expensive to do, as you have to pay for the annual storage costs as well as the harvesting costs should you need them – it's definitely a big commitment and consideration. Then once you're committed, how do you ever make the decision to throw the cord away? I'm only telling you about it because the service exists and if you are in a financial position to consider it, it's worth doing your own research and looking at your family's medical history – it could make a huge difference.

Apgar score To assess your baby's wellbeing, how she's reacting to the outside world, and whether she needs any extra medical attention, within the first minute of being born, and again at five minutes, the midwife will give her an Apgar test. Apgar stands for:

- **A**ctivity (muscle tone and movement)
- **P**ulse (heart rate)
- **G**rimace (reflex response)
- **A**ppearance (colour)
- **R**espiration (breathing)

Your baby will be given a score of 0, 1 or 2 for each of the five checks, so there's a maximum score of 10. A good healthy score is 7–10; a score of 4–6 might mean your baby needs some breathing assistance; a score of 3 or less might indicate your baby needs immediate medical assistance or resuscitation. Grading your newborn in the first minute of life is the fastest way to check her wellbeing and get help if needed. It's quite normal for Caesarean or premature babies to have a low Apgar score at the first-minute test.

When Belle was born, because she was five weeks premature, I'd been warned that she might have to go straight into an incubator, but when her checks came out well they passed her straight to me, which was amazing. However, after five minutes she turned blue, so the midwife put her under a heat lamp, where she stayed for 20 minutes to bring her temperature back up. The blue tone soon disappeared and she looked flushed and warm.

Within the first five minutes …

Further health checks In addition to the Apgar test, your midwife will probably use a suction bulb to clear your baby's nasal passages to aid breathing – particularly if it was a Caesarean birth. If your baby hasn't arrived through the birth canal and had all the mucus squeezed out en route, it is crucial to clear those channels. The midwife might give eyedrops as your baby's eyes will be sensitive to her new world. Think how you feel when you accidentally switch the bathroom light on during the night and then imagine not having been exposed to light before … ever! Your baby's vital first measurements – weight, length and head circumference – will be checked. These are the starting point of your baby's development and are crucial to track her ongoing progress. Your baby will be dried then wrapped in whatever outfit you brought along – unless she comes out so huge, or in my case with Belle so tiny, that nothing fits and you have to dispatch someone to the nearest baby clothing shop!

Within the first 24 hours …

Vitamin K injection Vitamin K is essential for blood clotting but babies are born with almost none in their system. To prevent a very rare blood disorder called Vitamin K Deficiency Bleeding (VKDB), the NHS recommends all newborns have a Vitamin K injection. If you're not keen on your baby having an injection, it can be given by mouth. If your baby is breastfed, it's three doses in total, two in the first week and the third when he's a month old. If your baby is bottle-fed, only the two doses in week one are necessary because there is Vitamin K in formula. I opted for the injection for all my children as I didn't trust myself to give it at the right times, and I know I would have worried about them vomiting it out after a feed. But the decision is completely up to you.

Within the first 72 hours …

Newborn and Infant Physical Examination (NIPE) Tests can vary between hospitals, but the NHS offers every baby a Newborn and Infant Physical Examination (NIPE) – even if you had a home birth. A healthcare professional will get a general overview from you about how your baby is feeding, whether she's producing plenty of nappies and how responsive she is. Then there will be a thorough health check: your baby's eyes will be examined to check for good movement and for conditions such as cataracts; her heart will be listened to for any irregularities; her hips checked for restricted movement; and with boys the testicles will be checked for any potential issues with them descending (they descend in the first few months after birth).

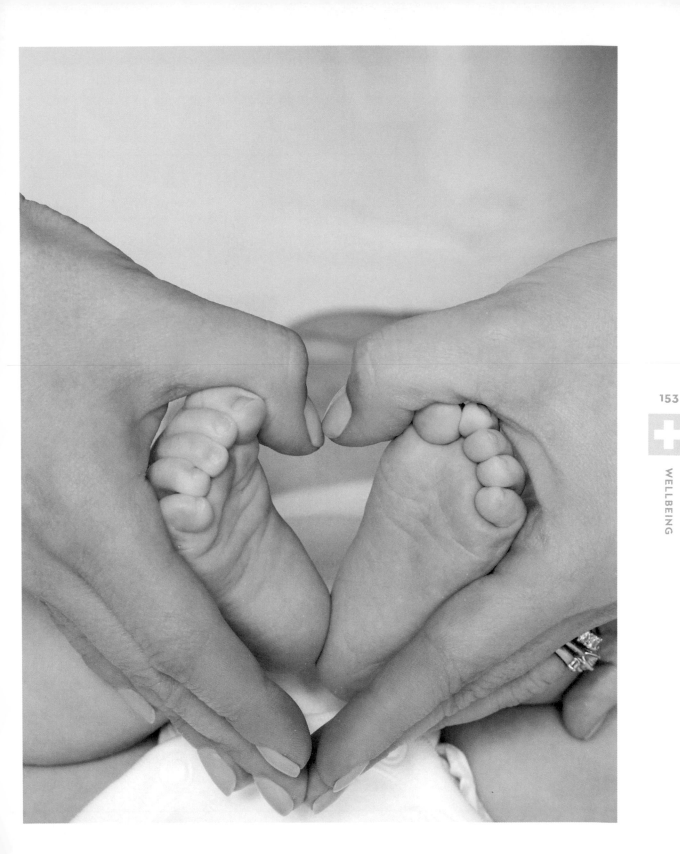

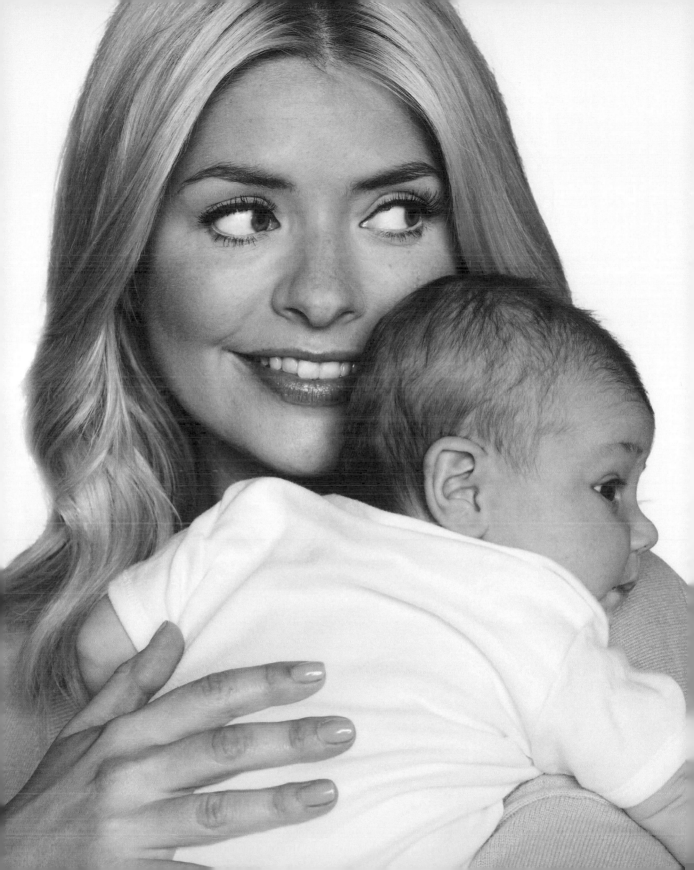

The red book All notes will be recorded in your baby's red Personal Child Health Record book. Keep this safe and take it to all of your baby's medical appointments. It will keep track of her progress and record any vaccinations for the first year and beyond.

Blood spot test Often referred to as the heel prick test, this rules out certain conditions, including sickle cell disease and cystic fibrosis. It takes a second for the midwife to prick your baby's heel to get a sample of four drops of blood. I don't think it hurts too much, especially if you make sure you're cuddling or feeding your baby whilst it's being done. Trust me, it's far worse for you watching, but it's far better to know about any serious conditions early on so that they can be acted on quickly. The results will come through the post around six weeks later, but if the test is positive you will be notified earlier.

Newborn hearing test The NHS offers every baby an Otoacoustic Emissions (OAE) test, often whilst you're still in hospital or in the first three months. A soft earpiece will be put in your baby's ear which plays clicking sounds to check that the inner ear (cochlea) is responding as it should. It doesn't hurt, and if all is well you'll be given the results straight away.

For an accurate reading, conditions need to be fairly perfect, so don't be alarmed if the test has to be repeated. Your baby being fractious or a noisy environment can affect the result, as can your baby having something, such as water, in her ear that temporarily blocks the signal. The OAE test may be repeated or a slightly different one, an AABR (Automated Auditory Brainstem Response) test, may be done. This involves little sensors being attached to your baby's head and headphones put over her ears.

You can decide whether to let your baby have these checks, but bear in mind that undetected hearing problems affect language and speech development, so it's important to discover them early on. Chester's hearing test suggested issues in one ear, which the doctors thought may have been because he arrived back to back (not the ideal position, as his back lay against my back) and it was a bit of a mission to deliver him! They thought his ears might have got blocked with fluid on the way out or from the birthing pool. However, on repeating the test three days later, all was fine.

Within the first week ...

Leaving hospital How long you stay in hospital really depends on what kind of delivery you had and whether it's your first baby. Hospitals are obviously keen to get you moving if all's well, but won't let you go until you are all in agreement you are ready. The average stay for a vaginal birth can vary; you might leave on the same day or stay in for two, and it'll probably be longer if you've had a Caesarean. The bottom line is don't go home until you are ready to. Use the expertise and support at the hospital to get you and your baby on your feet, particularly if you've had a difficult delivery.

Let's all take a moment to metaphorically high-five the Duchess of Cambridge, who brought her new baby, Princess Charlotte, out to meet the world's press less than twelve hours after giving birth. This just shows you how ready your body actually is for childbirth when the time comes. My mum's just informed me she was up, showered and with a full face of make-up, ready to receive hospital visitors within three hours of delivering me! I, on the other hand, minutes after having Harry, can remember Dan coming in to tell me he'd just bumped into Tess Daly and Vernon Kay in the corridor having their own tour of the maternity unit. So I, in my adrenalin-fuelled postpartum euphoria, suggested he invite them in to meet the baby. Thank goodness one of us was thinking straight – thank you, Daniel – as he quite rightly pointed out that it might not be the best time given the doctor was still stitching up my vagina! Half an hour later I got up to take a shower and passed out. My advice here is to take it slow! Kate Middleton, we salute you!

Visits from midwives Once you are home you will have several midwife visits (how many depends on how well you and your baby are doing at home). These visits are not to assess how clean and tidy your house is or whether your hair is greasy! They are primarily to check that you're all adapting well to life together at home and to assess the wellbeing of you and your baby. It's also your opportunity to ask any questions or get some extra help with breastfeeding if you're struggling, so don't be afraid to voice your concerns; the midwife will have heard them a dozen times before.

I had an interesting moment with my midwife – there's no advice in this story, but it might make you smile! When the first midwife turned up she was very beautiful and very young, and she suggested that because my records showed that I'd had an episiotomy she would need to do a full check.

We chatted for a good 15–20 minutes before she asked me to pop on the bed and lift my ankles above my head, which is no mean feat at the best of times, let alone four days after childbirth! It was at this opportune moment that she decided to tell me that we'd met before. I immediately thought, 'Oh gosh, she thinks she knows me because she recognises my face, but hasn't put two and two together because all my medical records are in my married name, not Willoughby.' But then she said, 'You've interviewed me ... I was in the pop group The Honeyz.' In one way, having my bum in the air served the purpose, eclipsing my very red face, but on the other hand, as you can imagine, I was mortified. Needless to say the chances of a 90s popstar arriving to check your stitches are minimal, so hopefully you'll have a better experience!

After the first week ...

The midwife visits usually stop when your baby is about ten days old, and then your health visitor will take over. Your health visitor is essentially a midwife and nurse combined, and will be your first point of contact on all the types of care your baby may need, physical, emotional and medical.

There are some things you'll need to be aware of, like the fact that you will have to take your baby to be weighed and measured at your nearest baby clinic and you have to book your baby in for her first immunisations (you'll be prompted to do so by your GP surgery), most of which happen in the first year (see pages 160–1). You'll also have your postpartum check six weeks after giving birth. During this appointment your GP will give your baby the once over, check your weight and blood pressure and take a urine sample. Depending on what kind of delivery you had, you might be offered an examination to check any stitches or your Caesarean scar. You'll also talk about contraception and your general emotional wellbeing, so use this opportunity to ask for help or discuss anything unusual you are experiencing or feeling.

02 Caring for your baby

Now this is where it all gets a bit personal. What your baby produces in her nappy can be a little odd, so whilst this isn't a particularly glamorous section, you'd rather know than not, right?! It's not all about poo though, I promise! You'll also find tips on how to bath your baby, how to get her through teething and how to babyproof the house.

There are also some important medical appointments you need to schedule for your baby by way of vaccinations to make sure that she's protected from a young age. Healthwise, your first instinct when your baby shows signs of illness that you don't recognise will be to call the doctor, which is completely natural and you should absolutely follow your gut instinct. I'm not here to say when you shouldn't seek medical attention for your baby, but I have tried to give you examples of when you most definitely should and some serious symptoms you should be able to recognise.

There's no two ways about it, caring for your baby is a big responsibility, but you already have most of the tools you need instinctively to do the best job you can! I promise!

BABY CLINIC

After the first couple of weeks, you'll only need to take your baby to be weighed and measured about once a month, unless told otherwise. Her progress will be recorded in her red book on a centile chart. Boys and girls have different charts as they tend to grow at different rates. The most important thing to remember with this centile chart, as I mentioned in the Feeding chapter, is not whether your baby is on the 40th or 100th percentile, but whether she continues to grow at a continuous rate. So alarm bells should only start to ring if your baby is on the 100th one month and then on the 30th the next visit. The charts are just a guide to help everyone plot your baby's development and keep an eye on any potential health issues.

Harry was your classic bouncing baby, getting chubbier by the week and always top of the percentile chart, to the point where I actually stopped taking him to be weighed after a couple of months because I could see with my own eyes that he was progressing well. Having been born at just over 5lb (just over 2kg), I'm happy and proud to say that Belle caught up with the other full-term babies very quickly, so there were no problems there. Chester, on the other hand, was a complete nightmare. He'd gain weight one week, lose weight the next, and I ended up buying my own baby-weighing scales so I could keep an eye on him at home. At my lowest point I was weighing him before and after feeds – which is not to be recommended – but at that time I was doing anything to make myself feel better.

Go prepared Your baby will have to be naked at weigh-in, so make sure you take a spare nappy with you to put on her afterwards. It's also a good idea to take a clean muslin to lay your baby on because the weighing scales are always cold. Dress your baby in something that's really easy to take off and put on again, as there will be a hundred other mothers in the room and you'll inevitably feel like all those eyes are judging how adept you are with your child!

VACCINATIONS

We are very lucky in the UK to be offered all our baby's vaccinations on the NHS. In my view it's crucial to find out what's on offer and give your baby the best protection available.

Vaccinations are invariably administered into your baby's thigh. I won't lie, it's a bit traumatic to sit through your little bundle of joy being jabbed with a needle, but I think it's worse for you as you know what's coming. Your baby will have no idea until it's over (or until she gets a bit older) and will be fine as long as you hold her close.

Always make sure your baby is in good health before you take her for a vaccination. If she has a high temperature, phone and postpone until she is well. Having a high temperature is the body's way of fighting an existing infection, so it's definitely not the time to throw any more foreign antibodies into the mix. After a vaccination your baby might get a fever and the skin around the injection site will become red and slightly swollen. There are conflicting views on whether you should use infant paracetamol as a preventative measure, or wait until she presents a fever, but vaccinations don't happen very often and I always thought it was better not to let them get as far as a fever. I always gave mine infant paracetamol afterwards, which is permitted from two months (you have to wait at least 20 minutes after an injection), just to try to get ahead of the game. If they then became really poorly, I'd follow the dosage guidelines for the rest of the day.

Something which I have heard about – but I must stress is extraordinarily rare – is that a child might have a fit following a vaccination, in which case call an ambulance immediately. This would probably happen straight afterwards, when you're still with the nurse, but if you are on your own, put your baby in the recovery position (on her side) and count how many seconds she fits for so that you can tell the paramedics.

> I breastfed or bottle-fed my babies during their jabs to give them something nicer to think about!

1ST VACCINATION: ON DAY 1 ...

VITAMIN K: Within the first 24 hours, your baby will be offered a Vitamin K injection or oral suspension, which helps the blood clot so your baby doesn't get any internal bleeding. This is a very rare condition but it's worth it to eliminate the risk altogether. Depending on where you live and the risk of your child getting tuberculosis (TB), your baby might be offered a BCG vaccine.

2ND ROUND OF VACCINATIONS: AT 8 WEEKS ...

THE 5-IN-1 VACCINE: This is one injection that protects against diphtheria, whooping cough, polio, tetanus and Haemophilus influenzae type B (Hib is a bacterial infection that can lead to pneumonia and one type of meningitis).

THE PNEUMOCOCCAL VACCINE (PCV): This is another injection that protects against pneumonia, meningitis and septicaemia.

THE ROTAVIRUS VACCINE: This is a liquid vaccine that is given to your baby to swallow and protects against the rotavirus infection, which causes diarrhoea and vomiting and can be dangerous for a baby.

MEN B VACCINE: This injection also protects against meningitis, but the meningococcal group B bacterial strain.

3RD ROUND OF VACCINATIONS: AT 12 WEEKS ...

THE 5-IN-1 VACCINE: Booster dose.

MEN C VACCINE: This injection also protects against meningitis, but the meningococcal group C bacterial strain.

THE ROTAVIRUS VACCINE: Booster dose.

4TH ROUND OF VACCINATIONS: AT 16 WEEKS ...

THE 5-IN-1 VACCINE: Booster dose.

THE PNEUMOCOCCAL VACCINE (PCV): Booster dose.

MEN B VACCINE: Booster dose.

5TH ROUND OF VACCINATIONS: AT 12 MONTHS ...

HIB/MEN C VACCINE: This is given as one injection containing the meningitis C booster vaccine and the fourth Hib dose.

MEASLES, MUMPS AND RUBELLA VACCINE (MMR): One injection to protect against all three diseases.

THE PNEUMOCOCCAL VACCINE (PCV): Second booster dose.

MEN B VACCINE: Second booster dose.

SOME MEDICAL ADVICE

When to call for help ...

Babies frequently get a high temperature as it's their body's way of fighting any foreign nasties lurking within, and most of the time you can bring it down with regular doses of infant paracetamol. You can call the NHS non-emergency helpline any time for advice, call your health visitor or speak to your local pharmacist. However, babies are so little and their immune systems so immature, they can often go downhill quite quickly – so if your gut instinct is telling you to seek urgent medical help, then do it. It's not worth hesitating. I've listed below when symptoms would have become serious enough for me to call 999 for an ambulance.

- **High temperature:** If your baby is under a year old and has a high temperature of 40°C/104°F or more.
- **Dehydration:** Was your baby's last wet nappy over six hours ago? Does she have a dry tongue and lips? Is she floppy? Does the fontanelle (see opposite) look sunken or raised/bulging?
- **Vomiting:** Has your baby been continuously sick until there's nothing left in her system to come up but yellow/green bile? Is she vomiting blood?
- **Unusual nappy content:** Has your baby produced a black/red colour nappy meaning there is blood in her poo? Does your baby have blood in her nappy or little orangey-pink crystals, which could be a sign of dehydration?
- **Unusual rash:** Does your baby have a rash that won't disappear if you press a glass to it? This could be a symptom of meningitis.
- **Whooping cough:** Does your baby have a dreadful cough and is she gasping for air in between bouts? This could be whooping cough, so get it checked out.
- **Breathing difficulties:** Does she have a blue tinge to her skin? Is your baby wheezy or grunting? Is she breathing overly fast or does her chest seem to heave and suck right in when she breathes? Harry was really poorly once and when I took him to the doctor he was diagnosed with baby bronchiolitis. Being my first baby and the first time he had

something wrong, I sat with him all night to watch him breathing. You feel really hopeless when they're ill, but babies are tougher than they look.

- Floppiness: Is your baby floppy and unresponsive? This can be a sign of something more serious, such as meningitis, so seek medical advice, particularly if it's accompanied by a high fever.
- Raised or sunken fontanelle: This is the soft bit on top of a baby's head where the skull bone hasn't yet fused together, to allow your baby to pass through the birth canal more easily. If the fontanelle is raised or bulging, it can be a sign of inflammation, and if it's sunken, it's a symptom of extreme dehydration.

Basic first aid ...

I strongly recommend you attend some sort of first-aid course to learn the basics should the unthinkable happen with your baby. You will learn techniques such as the recovery position and how to help a choking child. If you have the time and the inclination, you never know when such knowledge might come in useful to help your family or someone else's.

Storing and giving medicines ...

I always keep the children's medicines in the fridge for safety, but check the packaging in case this contradicts storage recommendations. Most bottled liquids come with plastic syringes, which are brilliant for getting medicine into your child. Try to point it at an angle, into their cheek rather than straight down their throat. I tried it on myself with some of my cough medicine and nearly choked – mind you, babies don't have a gag reflex so they're probably all right if you shoot it straight down. Less chance of them being able to spit it out!

Giving eyedrops If you have to give your child eyedrops, drop them onto your baby's closed lids, then when she opens them the drops will trickle into the right spot.

Cranial osteopathy ...

Cranial osteopathy can help to release tension in a baby after birth through targeted massage. A baby's cranium responds quickly to osteopathy, and this treatment is particularly effective for babies who had a difficult birth, are colicky and those born by Caesarean. Being born suddenly by Caesarean can be quite a shock for babies, leaving them with tension in both their heads and their tummies that can be relieved by a cranial osteopath. The area of tension in the cranium is released by gentle physical manipulation, encouraging the body's own healing mechanism. Through gentle stretching and massage, it can release things like trapped wind in a colicky baby and promote general health and wellbeing.

Harry was a forceps baby. I didn't know enough about cranial osteopathy at the time, but I took him as soon as a friend told me about it. Even though he was much older, I really felt it made a difference. I took Chester because he was a reflux baby and delivered back to back, and I definitely think it helped. Check with your GP before taking your baby and then find a registered practitioner.

NAPPIES

Let's talk nappies! Which ones should you use? How many wet/dirty nappies should your baby have in a day? And what will you find in them?! I know – delightful! If you're reading this before your baby arrives, it might seem inconceivable that there should be so much to say and, more importantly, so much interest in what's in a baby's nappy. But believe me when I say it will become an obsession shared by you and your fellow mummies! So here goes!

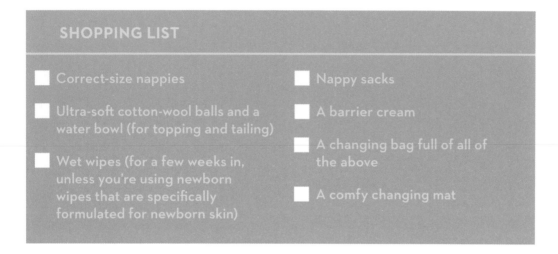

SHOPPING LIST

- ☐ Correct-size nappies
- ☐ Ultra-soft cotton-wool balls and a water bowl (for topping and tailing)
- ☐ Wet wipes (for a few weeks in, unless you're using newborn wipes that are specifically formulated for newborn skin)
- ☐ Nappy sacks
- ☐ A barrier cream
- ☐ A changing bag full of all of the above
- ☐ A comfy changing mat

Disposable v. reusable …

If your quandary is based on which nappies are cheaper and kinder to the environment then reusables might seem like the friendlier option. However, you'll need to do your research and sums to get an accurate comparison. It might seem criminal throwing out a nappy every few hours, which is going to take years to decompose at your nearest landfill site, but don't forget how much energy and water you'll be using at home to clean the reusable ones. You'll need to know how efficient your washing machine is and also consider whether you'll be tumble-drying them before you can work out what the best decision is for you.

Reusable nappies come in two types: two-part nappies, which have a material layer against the skin and a waterproof layer over it; and all-in-one nappies, which resemble disposable nappies and are bulky, so slow to dry out. If you do want to go down the reusable route but want to make it as easy as possible for yourself in terms of cleaning and drying the nappies, then there are plenty of useful sites online that will help you to find a service in your area.

You can also buy biodegradable 'eco' nappies and nappy sacks, which are more environmentally friendly than normal disposable nappies. They also have fewer chemicals and no bleaching agents, if you're worried about that. You should do your own research on this as they are more expensive than other disposables and, as far as I can tell, don't completely biodegrade, so it's completely up to you what you choose.

In the name of modern-mum convenience, I used disposable nappies for all of mine. For me, there's more than enough laundry piling up with a new baby without throwing a load of dirty nappies into the mix. And the thought of waiting for a bucket of dirty nappies to be full enough to put a wash on only served to seal the deal in my mind. All of my children were in nappies until they were about two and a half, and even longer if you count the night-time nappies.

Beware the nappy mountain! …

I can remember being surprised at how quickly that enormous basket of nappies I'd lovingly stacked during pregnancy disappeared without a trace! However many you've bought in preparation, know that you're going to need so many more, but actually I wouldn't do the big stock-up until after your baby is born. You can hazard a guess and go for the national average first-size nappy, which I did very successfully with Harry, who arrived a healthy 7lb (3kg). But when I did the same in preparation for Belle, who arrived five weeks early weighing just over 5lb (2kg), it was weeks before she was in those same newborn nappies. They swamped her, as did all the newborn-size clothes I'd bought.

Remember that babies grow really quickly at the start, so even if you got lucky and bought the correct size, you don't want to be left with 100 nappies you can't use because your baby is too small. It's a case of little and often when it comes to nappy shopping in the early days, I'm afraid.

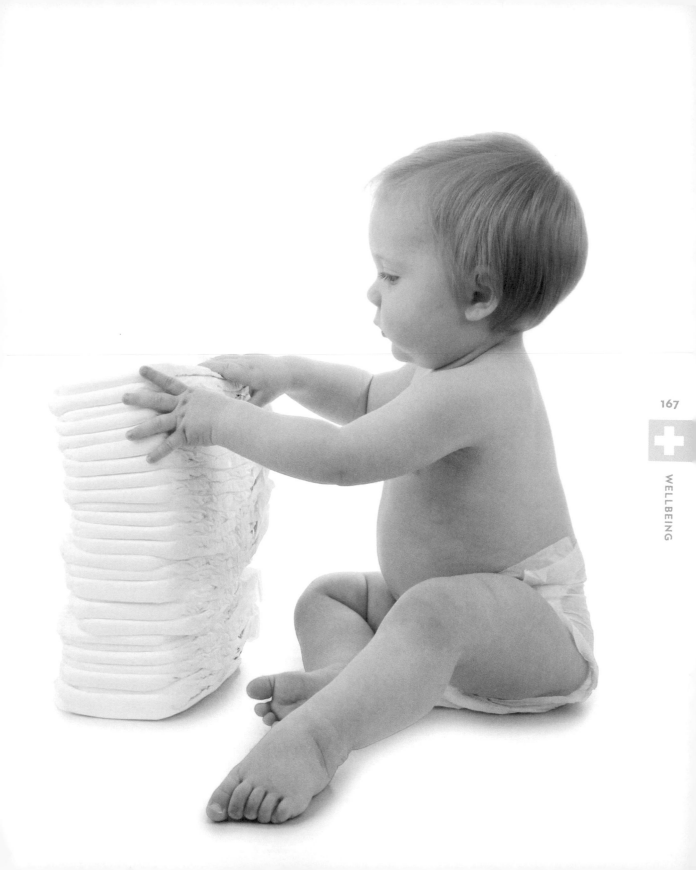

The nappy-changing headlines ...

FOR BABY BOYS

- I don't know what it is about little boys, but you can guarantee as soon as you open their nappy they decide to have a wee. There's something about the fresh air hitting their bits that brings it on. The only advice I can give here is to be ready with a muslin or something to intercept the spray! Luckily it's something they grow out of as the months go by!
- Remember to point his penis directly downwards into the nappy, or when he tiddles it will come out the top of the nappy.
- Despite all the bits being on the outside, which is easier in a way, you have to make sure you move everything around (gently) and check underneath to make sure you clean everywhere. Don't push back the foreskin when cleaning.

FOR BABY GIRLS

- It's very important to wipe from front to back so that you don't transfer any bottom bacteria to the vaginal area. Don't attempt to clean inside the vagina.
- It's not uncommon for girls to get a little bloodstain in her nappy, called a false menstruation, which is a result of your hormones running through her system and nothing at all to worry about.

FOR BOTH

- Watch out for the umbilical cord! When changing a newborn, always remember to fold the nappy down over the tabs to make sure the umbilical cord is left clear and not caught up inside. It's a good idea to check how the stump looks every time you change your baby's nappy until it drops off. To keep it clean, use some cooled, boiled water and gently wipe around the base with some soft cotton wool. If you think the area looks infected, i.e. it is red, seeping or smelly, then contact your midwife or GP right away.

Hygiene! Always wash your hands after changing a nappy. It sounds obvious, but all it takes is a microscopic bit of poo to be transferred from your hand to your baby's mouth for her to be at risk of getting a serious infection.

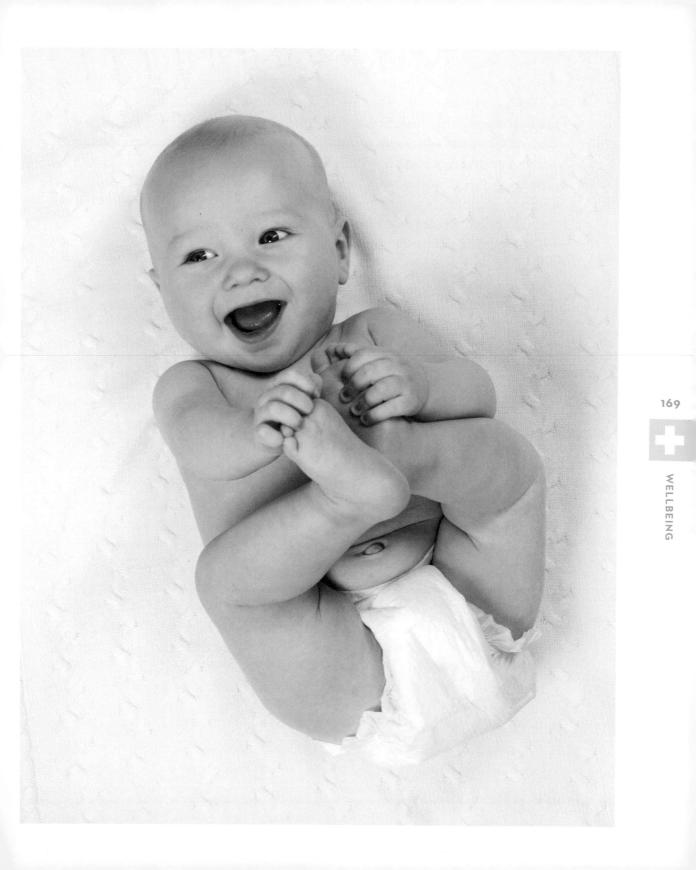

How to: clean your baby's bottom ...

Newborn skin is very delicate, so it's best to just use cotton wool and cooled, boiled water to wipe your baby clean (see topping and tailing, pages 178–9) unless you buy the ultra-gentle newborn wet wipes. I always found it useful to use the nappy for the first wipe using a firm downward motion. When you move to wipes, I'd recommend unperfumed ones. Make sure your baby's bottom is clean and dry before applying a thin layer of barrier cream to prevent nappy rash. Babies have so many creases, so be really thorough, checking up their back too for anything that might have escaped! This attention to detail and using a good barrier cream really is your only guard against nappy rash (see below).

Nappy rash ...

Nappy rash is caused by the bacteria in your baby's bowel movements turning into ammonia, which aggravates delicate skin. It can vary from a bit of redness to weeping sores, which are heartbreaking for you to discover but will heal with some care. Treat it with a barrier cream as soon as you see it.

With Harry, a stronger metanium ointment was the only thing that made a difference. Just as a baby's skin heals quickly, it can deteriorate dramatically between nappy changes if you don't gently clean the area and cover it in cream. If it's really bad, avoid using baby wipes and go back to using cotton wool and cooled boiled water. As much as it pains your baby when you clean the area, you have to get rid of the bacteria. Once completely clean, slather on the cream to prevent the skin coming into direct contact with the nappy contents.

Nappy-off time I'm a big believer in giving your baby some nappy-free time to let her bottom 'breathe', as my mum always used to say. Imagine if you had a damp nappy clinging to you, day in, day out. It must feel so liberating to have a kick about without it and let the air get to the skin.

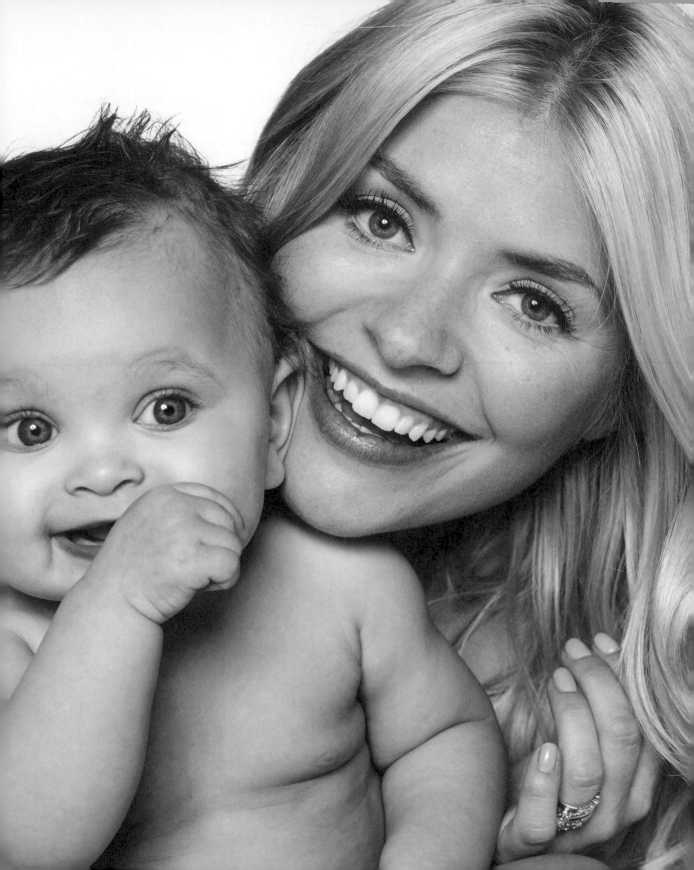

Watch out for the rolling baby …

Never leave a baby unattended on a changing table. When you're changing your baby and discover halfway through that you've run out of wipes, there's always a temptation to look down at your baby and say, 'Now you stay there, I'll be two seconds,' as you make a mad dash for the bathroom. And all might be well but, believe me, your baby can develop a new movement overnight and, before you know it, will have decided to choose that moment to roll over for the first time – a metre off the floor! Not leaving your baby unattended is a good habit to get into from the start. It's just not worth the risk.

If you have a wriggler on your hands, which all babies go through in that first year, you might find it easier to change her on a towel on the floor so you have more room to manoeuvre. It's also an idea to give her something to hold – a toy or anything you have handy. Even the wet-wipe packet can be like the eighth wonder of the world to your curious little mover! If you don't have anything to hold her interest, just talking and making faces can be enough to entertain her! I used to give my children a plastic mirror to hold, as their own reflection seemed to stop them in their tracks!

How many, and what looks normal? …

A newborn might go through up to twelve nappies a day, especially if she is feeding well. This will slowly reduce as your baby's digestion system and kidneys become more developed and her feeding routine more established. By about four weeks you might only be getting through about eight nappies a day, and the majority of these will be just wet. As the weeks go by, babies are all different in terms of how often they poo and you can get obsessed with when they last went. As gross as it sounds, it's important to keep half an eye on what sort of nappies you're getting and how often. As I said, nappy contents are an excellent way of tracking your baby's health, so here are some helpful notes for you and your newborn. As a general rule, as long as you're getting plenty of wet nappies and when you do get a dirty one, the poo – whatever the colour – is soft, your baby is doing well.

Baby's first week of nappies …

DAYS 1–2: On average 2+ wet nappies and 1+ dirty nappy per day …	Green-brown-black sticky poo. **Your baby's first poo is called meconium. Surprisingly, it doesn't look anything like you would expect – it's more like tar than poo! But the good news is it doesn't really smell of anything and is a by-product of all the mucus your baby digested in the womb.**
DAYS 3–4: On average 3+ wet nappies and 2+ dirty nappies per day …	Poo that's more green/brown than black. **As your baby feeds and the milk passes through her digestive system, the colour of the poo will change and at this stage it's more greeny/brown than black and sticky.**
DAYS 5–6: On average 5+ wet nappies and 2+ dirty nappies per day …	Mustard-yellow poo. **By now, if your baby is feeding well, the colour of the poo will change to a bright mustard yellow if you're breastfeeding and slightly browner if you're formula-feeding. This is a great sign, and means that your baby's system is running well and that all the meconium has gone.**

After the first week …

Once your baby is pooping mustard three or more times a day and giving you five or more wet nappies, you're good to go. By this point you'll know what normal looks like, so just be aware if anything changes.

Poo check! You don't need to open a nappy every time to check if there's a poo, just pull at the leg elastic and have a quick peek!

TROUBLESHOOT:
NAPPY CONTENTS

Dark urine: Your baby's wet nappies should be colourless and odourless, so if you notice a dark yellow wet nappy or if you're hardly getting any wet nappies during the day, your baby could be dehydrated. Disposable nappies are very absorbent, so it can be difficult to tell how much urine your baby has passed – you could put tissue in the nappy to show it up. Some nappies have an indicator line inside that goes darker when they absorb fluid. If you have any dehydration concerns, contact your GP.

Urate crystals: These are tiny red/orange crystals that you might find in your baby's nappy in the first few days. These can be a sign that your baby is a bit dehydrated whilst you're both getting to grips with feeding. Don't panic, it's perfectly normal, but it's worth mentioning to your midwife if you do come across this scary little red stain in your baby's nappy.

Green poo: If your baby's stools don't ever turn mustard yellow and are green, it is often a result of a breastfeeding baby not getting to the hindmilk (see page 24). If she's only getting the lactose-packed foremilk, then you might find she's producing green poo and is slow to gain weight. Definitely speak to a medical professional if you're getting green nappies. If the green stools are accompanied by a fever or your baby's being sick, it can also signify some kind of infection in the gut and you should get medical advice straight away.

White-cream poo: A creamy white nappy can be a sign of a liver problem, so definitely take your baby to the GP. It's worth taking the nappy with you so that the doctor can see it and take a sample.

Blood: More often than not, it's nothing to worry about and may be the result of blood digested from your cracked nipples or, if your baby has been constipated, she might have a little tear in her bottom that is bleeding. When there is blood always see a medical professional to eliminate anything more serious.

Constipation ...

Formula-fed babies tend to get constipated more often than breastfed babies because formula doesn't contain the same hormones as breast milk, which help the gut break everything down. If your baby is straining and her poo comes out in hard, dry 'rabbit droppings', she's constipated. But if she's straining and the poo is soft, she's fine. Most babies strain and go red when they poo.

All babies go through phases of being constipated and some might not poo for a week. It won't do them any harm, but might make them a bit tetchy! There are little tricks you can use to help them if you are really worried, like putting a couple of drops of orange juice and water in one of the medicine pipettes and giving it to them that way. I would never have done this with Chester, though, because the acid would only have aggravated his reflux. You can also try massaging the tummy in light clockwise circular movements to encourage bowel movement. Syrup of figs is another solution you can get at the chemist, but if you are really concerned, speak to your GP who may prescribe something.

Explosive nappies (be prepared!) ...

I don't know any mother who hasn't been caught short by an explosive nappy. It's normal for babies to have runny stools because of all the milk, so always have at least one change of clothes in your changing bag when you're out and about. You'd be amazed how far runny poo can travel up your baby's back. Delightful! It might be a two-man job just to get your baby out of her dirty clothes without covering the rest of her in it. Being prepared is your best defence! This is when you realise why it's good to have your own travel changing mat, rather than expose your baby to public ones. You can imagine the germs and bacterial infections you might pick up from unhygienic changing facilities.

If you're worried your baby might be unwell and that she has diarrhoea rather than just loose stools, take her to the GP. You'll often find that diarrhoea poo is much smellier and accompanied by a high temperature. You don't want your baby to get dehydrated, so feed her more often if you think this is the case.

WASHING YOUR BABY

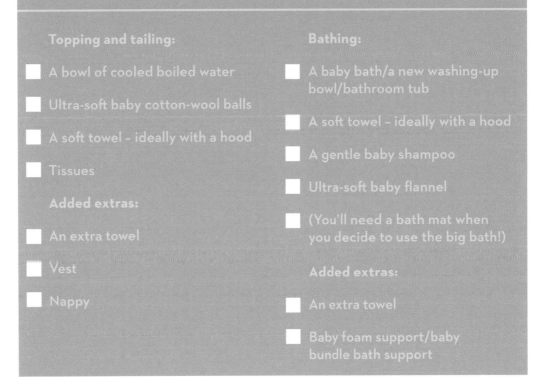

SHOPPING LIST

Topping and tailing:

☐ A bowl of cooled boiled water

☐ Ultra-soft baby cotton-wool balls

☐ A soft towel – ideally with a hood

☐ Tissues

Added extras:

☐ An extra towel

☐ Vest

☐ Nappy

Bathing:

☐ A baby bath/a new washing-up bowl/bathroom tub

☐ A soft towel – ideally with a hood

☐ A gentle baby shampoo

☐ Ultra-soft baby flannel

☐ (You'll need a bath mat when you decide to use the big bath!)

Added extras:

☐ An extra towel

☐ Baby foam support/baby bundle bath support

Bathtime = tantrum time! ...

For the first week or so you will probably just wash your baby every day by topping and tailing her, which I'll explain in a moment. But I'd like to start with a warning about a reaction you may not have expected – when the time comes to undress and lower your baby into her first proper bath I guarantee you'll never have heard screams or witnessed a meltdown like it! She's likely to be incandescent with rage the first few times, which can be daunting for any parent, so I would definitely recommend asking someone to help with bathtime until she settles down. It can be quite stressful trying to calm a red, shaking, chicken-legged, slippery little baby whilst grabbing for a towel and anything else out of reach without an extra pair of hands. There's a bit of a knack to holding a wet baby steady and safely in the bath, and to begin with

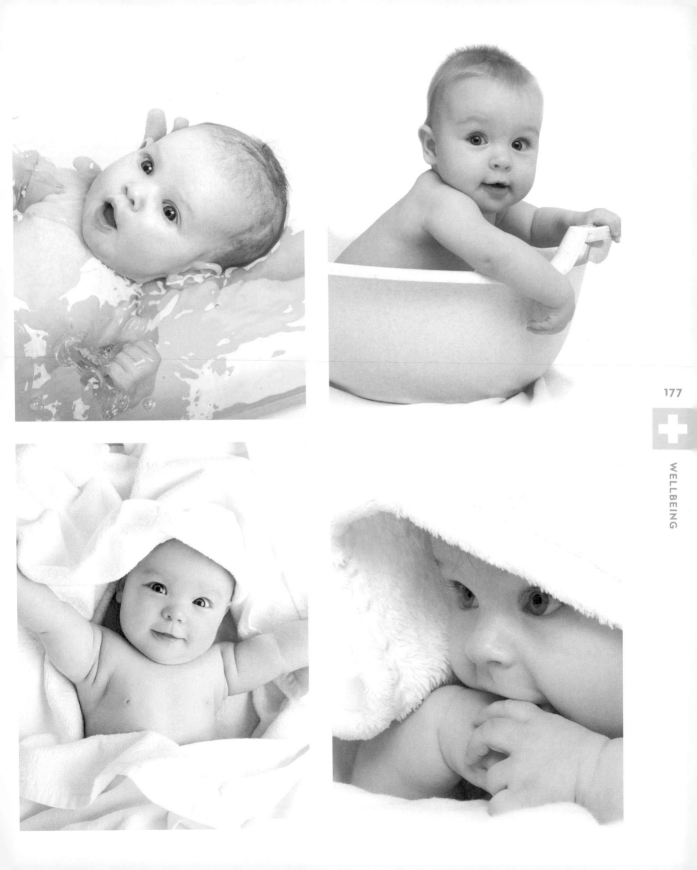

you might feel that this is an impossible job for one person. But don't get disheartened. Your baby won't always be this fed up at bathtime and you'll both get better with practice. Once she finally relaxes into it and realises how much she actually loves the sensation of the warm water on her skin, and the feel of your touch and sound of your voice as you wash her, it will soon become one of her favourite times of the day. Just think how wonderfully soothing you find slipping into a steaming bath after a long day!

Big bath v. baby bath ...

Harry and Belle never had a baby bath. They went straight into the big bath. I held them behind the neck and under the shoulders with one hand and sloshed water over them. They loved the freedom of being able to kick out freely. However, awkward chops, Chester, couldn't have been more different. He'd freak out in a big bath so first of all I started bathing with him and breastfeeding him in the bath but in the end I remember asking Dan to go out and buy a baby bath very late one evening. Chester loved the security of being in something with sides, with hindsight, the fact it was more snug and more upright made complete sense, given his reflux.

Time for bathtime If I can give you one piece of advice to make the early days easier, don't bath your baby straight after a feed or when she's hungry. Plan and pick a time in between feeds when she's at her most content, to give you both the best chance of a happy bathtime!

When and how to bath your baby safely ...

The first week Immediately after birth the midwife will clean your baby up as much as you want her to. Sometimes it's better to leave any vernix (see page 147) still present after birth as it acts as a moisturising, protective layer against her new environment.

I was told with all three of my babies that it wasn't necessary to fully bath them for the first week as it would dry out their sensitive skin, but it's completely up to you when you bath your baby. There are no hard-and-fast rules, just as long as you leave it until at least an hour after birth. You might be taught how to top and tail your baby whilst still in hospital, which essentially means learning how to clean her bottom, face and hands hygienically. If you're not, then ask your midwife to show you the safest way to do it once she visits you at home.

The most important thing to remember with topping and tailing is to use a new piece of cotton wool, dipped in a bowl of cooled boiled water for each wipe, to prevent the transfer of infection. I used to set up in a warm room and leave my babies in their vest and nappy whilst I did this so they didn't get chilly and feel completely exposed. Leave the poppers undone on the vest so you can get to the umbilical cord. I'd always recommend starting at the top, softly wiping your baby's eyes using a different ball for each eye, then I'd get another few balls to clean the rest of the face, being sure to do under the milk-encrusted chin and neck creases and behind the ears.

> A bath won't stop your baby's cord stump healing, but be very gentle with that area and dab it dry with a tissue, not a rough towel.

In the early days, steer clear of the insides of your baby's ears or you might do more damage than good. You can also wipe over the top of her head (whether she has hair or not) and hands. Then wrap the top end of your baby in a warm towel, and, using new cotton balls for every area, gently wash the base of the umbilical cord before patting it dry with a tissue. Clean your baby's genitals thoroughly; if you have a boy, avoid pulling the foreskin back, and with girls, don't try to clean inside the vagina and always wipe front to back.

Subsequent weeks When you feel ready to give your baby her first bath you'll need to be as organised as possible. Plan for every scenario and make sure you have everything you need to hand.

You want to do it where it is nice and warm, so maybe use a plastic bath placed securely on the kitchen table. You can of course put your baby straight into the big bath, but make sure you have a non-slip bath mat and also be aware that it will kill your back when they're really small – you have to be bent over and holding them firm the whole time. If you don't go for a baby bath, a new (clean) washing-up bowl will do. As soon as her limbs start poking out above the sides, you'll know it's time to move her up to the bathroom!

You don't have to bath your newborn daily. Every two or three days is fine, but just make sure you top and tail in between. It's important to keep bathing her, though, so she gets used to it and learns to love it. A bath might only last as long as a couple of minutes, so don't feel you have to make it last any longer than is comfortable for both of you. And I wouldn't use any baby washes or anything for the first month as your baby's skin is still so delicate. The aim is to just get her clean, which water will do very well.

When everything's ready, undress your baby, hold her close to make her feel secure and warm, and lower her in slowly so that she doesn't feel suddenly abandoned! You can actually wash her face, under her chin and behind her ears as you would if you were topping and tailing, before you even put her in the bath, so that's the top half dealt with already! Then, putting one hand under her bottom and the other around her shoulders, neck and head so she is well supported, slowly lower her in and let her get used to the warmth and sensation of the water. If you feel confident enough to let go of her bottom half, freeing up that hand to gently slosh some water over her, then great, but if not, get your washing wingman to do that bit. As I said, this only needs to last for as long as you both want it to, so as soon as you like, lift your baby out, wrap her up in a towel and give her a big, congratulatory cuddle. You'll have both earned it!

Water level and temperature ...

Keep the water at a fairly low level – no more than about 7cm/3in, so you don't end up with water pouring out over the sides once you've got your wriggly baby and both hands in! Get yourself a bath thermometer, if possible, to alleviate any doubt over water temperature. It will also tell you the temperature of the room before you put it into the bath. It's important to get the water temperature right as your baby won't appreciate a cold bath and it's dangerous to have it too hot. If you haven't got a thermometer, the old-school way of testing is to put your elbow in. You're looking for a temperature of 37–38°C (98.6–100.4°F), which is what your body temperature should be. A good tip to make sure you the water isn't too hot is to run the cold first, then warm it up.

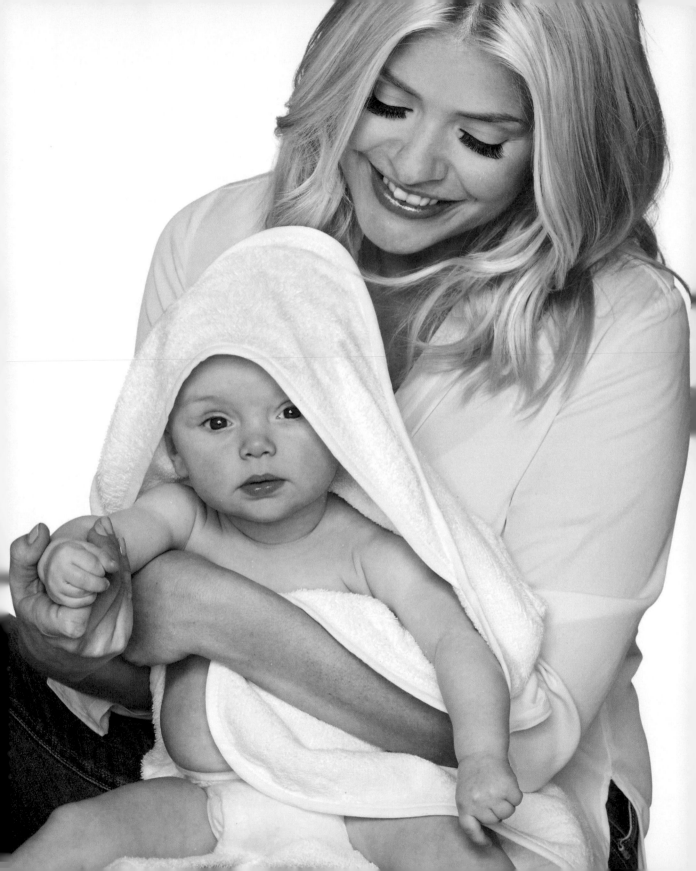

Bath aids ...

There are lots of things you can buy to make your baby's bathtime a more pleasurable experience for both of you. One of the simplest things to do when your baby is really little is to sink a flannel onto the bottom of the bath, as this is softer than a rubber mat. I tried a towelling baby support, which all of mine loved because you could lay them in it – think baby deckchair experience! – and they felt fully supported, with no slipping and sliding about in your arms. It also left me hands-free to stroke, wash and play with them, and because the support was made of fabric, the warm water comes through it, so they got a real sense of being submerged. Depending on which one you buy, you can also put the towelling part straight in the washing machine, so there's no chance of bacterial build-up. You can get a similar support with a foam bottom – a bit like a baby-size sponge mattress – which is really squidgy and comfy, but you have to make sure you dry it out properly after use to keep it hygienic. It goes without saying that you should never leave your child unattended in water, no matter how shallow – babies (and adults!) can drown in as little as 2½cm/1in of water. If you opt for a chair, remember that, whilst these give your baby independence, you should only use them if you are sure your baby is really ready and strong enough sitting upright without a tendency to topple over.

You don't need to buy bath toys for the first couple of months because your baby will be too young to play with them. Your touch and voice whilst she's in the bath is enough entertainment. Once she can sit unaided in the tub, toys can be a really fun addition.

Once your baby can sit up unaided, without toppling over, try a rubber bath mat that has a little seat coming out of it – or little bath seats that sucker to the bottom of the bath. I used one of these with Belle because I found it easier knowing that she was fully supported whilst I washed Harry. The chair was like an extra pair of hands when I was flying solo.

TROUBLESHOOT:
WHAT SHOULD I DO IF ...

▪ **My baby tiddles in the bath?** Babies will tiddle in the bath but it's not a health concern as urine is sterile and won't harm them – or you if you happen to be in with them!

▪ **My baby poos in the bath?** This has only happened with my children once, but the bottom line is, get them out quickly, deal with the offending matter, disinfect your bath and run another to wash your baby down thoroughly. On this particular occasion my child had an upset stomach and I don't think meant to poo. There have been other times where I've spotted them straining, so quickly got them out, dried them off and put a nappy on for them to continue! Oh, the glamour!

▪ **My baby hates the bath?** As I said, most babies hate bathtime to start with, but get used to it and learn to love it. The most likely factor is temperature – room temperature and/or bath temperature. I don't think a room can ever be too warm at bathtime for a naked baby but a bath can definitely be too cold or too hot. Also don't take too long over it. If your baby hates it, don't make it a long, drawn-out process that she dreads as soon as you start the routine. You could try getting in with your baby as it might be the separation she hates. You'll both enjoy going in together with all that skin-to-skin contact.

▪ **The unthinkable happens and my baby is scalded by hot bath water?** If this happens, phone the doctor immediately, or go to A&E if it's really serious. You should also cool the scalded area with lukewarm or cool water for 20 minutes, then cover the area with cling film and keep your baby warm whilst you're waiting for medical help. Thankfully, this has never happened to my children, as I'm paranoid about water temperature and always use my bath thermometer. Just be careful. Your baby's skin is thin and delicate and can't cope with extreme conditions, so you have to help her look after it.

My baby has cradle cap. Can I wash it? Cradle cap is when you see greasy yellow-brown scales on your baby's scalp, which you'll be tempted to peel off. Your baby's scalp is delicate so you don't want to do anything that's going to leave it feeling sore, sensitive or, worse, infected. The scales will eventually disappear on their own and are not at all painful for your baby – things like massaging olive or almond oil into the scalp at night, and washing with a cradle cap shampoo, can help the process. But, and I'm saying this with caution as it did turn out to be a miracle cure, when I had Chester a friend of mine told me to mix a teaspoon of bicarbonate of soda with water to form a paste and paint it on all the affected areas, so I did. On her recommendation I left it for five minutes and could see it lifting the cap, and then when I washed it off, all I can say is that it was the first old wives' tale I've heard that actually worked!

My baby shivers after a bath even when she's warm? Sometimes a baby will shiver or tremble, but it's not necessarily down to being cold. It can just be a result of her immature, underdeveloped nervous system and will stop when she's a few months old.

My baby gets bath water in her eyes? There's nothing wrong with this, other than your baby being taken by surprise and having a momentary meltdown. In fact, from about three months it's worth you getting your baby used to the feeling of having water in her eyes. If you get her used to it at this young age, it will build her confidence in and around water, which will stand her in great stead further down the line when she's learning to swim. From a really early age, Harry, Belle and Chester all had what started as a little bit of water being splashed in their eyes to full-on cups being poured over their hair as they got bigger. As long as you buy a tear-free shampoo, there's no reason not to get them used to having water in their eyes. I think the worst thing you can do is go out of your way for them not to experience this!

Baby massage ...

Massaging your baby can be one of the loveliest, most calming things for both of you. I always did this for mine in the bathroom, straight after the bath, where it's warm and, if possible, not too brightly lit. Below is a little routine to try, and you can also take classes (see page 228). Be guided by what your baby seems to be enjoying; she'll soon let you know which movements she likes.

- Begin on the arms or legs, with a little baby oil rubbed into your hands. Start at the top of each and firmly but gently pull downwards in one slow, smooth action, repeating a few times.
- When you've finished each leg, move on to her feet, using your thumbs to massage her soles in little circles (see photo 1, opposite). Do the same with the palm of each hand once you've finished her arms (see photo 2). You can also very gently tug on each finger and toe if you like.
- Move on to her chest, making little circular motions with your forefingers (see photo 3). If she's constipated you can also do this on her tummy, which can really help with her digestion.
- Follow this with some long strokes, starting just under her shoulder and tracing your fingers all the way down to her hip (see photo 4).
- If your baby likes being on her tummy you can make similar circular motions on her back, or long, steady strokes from her neck to her bottom.

Cutting your baby's nails ...

The first time you pick up safety nail scissors (the ones with the ball-shaped tips in case your baby flinches) can be very daunting. But you'll soon become a dab hand and get to the point where you'll feel like you're cutting your baby's nails every two minutes!

When your baby is very tiny you'll notice that her nails are paper-thin and almost just tear off, so you could give that a go, or bite them off gently with your teeth. It might sound weird, but your mouth is much more sensitive to feeling where the nails join the fingertips. If you use a pair of scissors from day dot, make sure you do it somewhere bright and try to pull the pads back, one by one, before you start to cut. Round off each corner so they're not left sharp, which will do more damage than not cutting them at all. If you find your baby is still accidentally scratching herself, you can buy her scratch mittens.

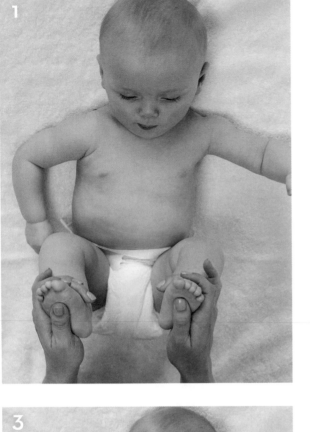

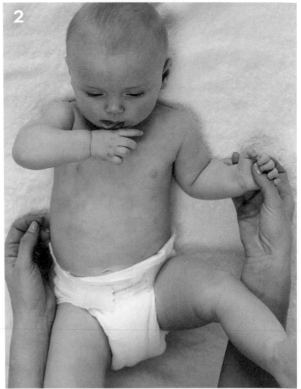

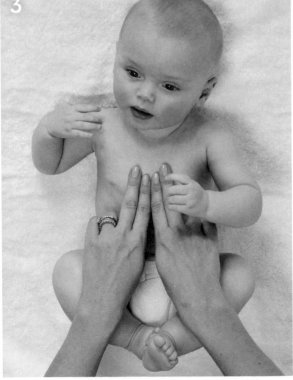

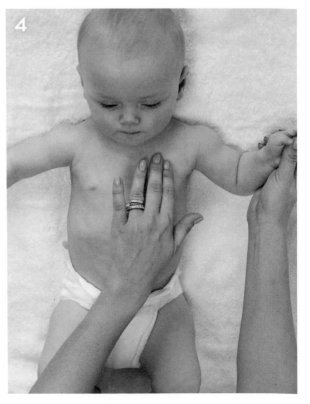

TEETHING

The teething phase can be one of the most challenging! It can start as early as three months or as late as twelve months, although the first tooth usually appears at around six. By about two years old, babies have 20 teeth in total and up to eight can arrive in the first year. Annoyingly, teething tends to flare up during the night, so you might have to relax the bedtime rules until that tooth arrives!

A teething baby is easy to spot: flushed cheeks; fever; sore bottom; excessive dribbling; red, swollen gums; desperate to put everything and anything in her mouth; generally whingey and emotional.

How to help ...

Your teething baby will be in pain – some suffer terribly in the build-up to the tooth appearing and some only in the hours before. There are lots of remedies on the market you can try. You can give her infant paracetamol and there are over-the-counter gels you rub on the gum that are very effective, but read the dosage instructions as some should only be applied every three hours. Make sure you also check any medicines you're using are age appropriate.

I used homeopathic teething granules with all of mine, but Belle in particular responded to them. It was like she knew they were going to help and she would open her mouth like a baby bird. The granules come in sachets and look like icing sugar – you pour them into your baby's mouth and they dissolve and coat the gums. You can also buy teething rings to keep in the fridge – chewing these can be extra soothing for your baby's burning gums.

Little dribbler Put a bit of Vaseline under your baby's chin to stop it getting sore.

When to start brushing ...

With all of mine I started brushing as soon as the first tooth appeared! You can get those rubber brushes you put on your finger, which are gentle on the gums. When they get a few more teeth you can buy soft first toothbrushes and age-appropriate toothpaste.

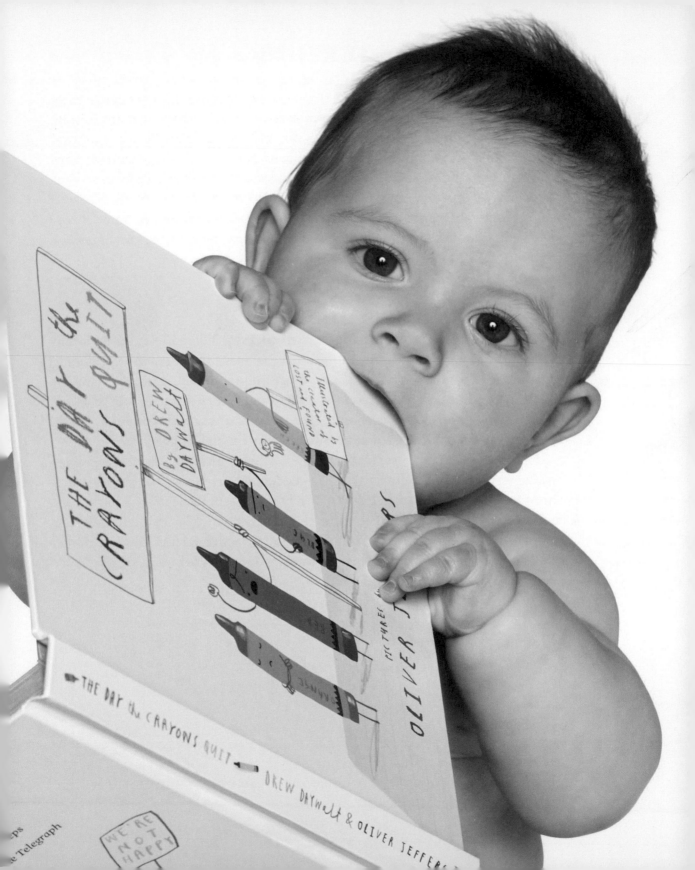

CRYING

Babies cry. It's what they do. They sleep, they eat and they cry! It's their only form of communication, so don't despair. The biggest challenge ahead of you is to listen to and learn about your baby's particular cries, recognising what they mean and finding out what soothes them. If you accept early on that there will be a few moments in the next year when nothing you do makes a darn bit of difference to stop your baby from crying, then you're one step ahead of the next mum, and mentally you won't be so hard on yourself. The real accomplishment here is learning how to cope in these moments and knowing that tomorrow is a new day!

It's worth mentioning here that when a baby cries a mother experiences the release of prolactin, which is essential for milk production, so is it any wonder you want to go running to any baby if you hear it in distress? Eventually you'll know your baby inside and out, and will be able to hear her cry in a room full of screaming children.

Crying in the first week ...

In the first few days babies don't really cry that much. In fact, they sleep and feed more than they cry, and just when you start to think how easy this all is, and how you've got the perfect child who never cries, she wakes up!

At this point no new mother on the planet will know what her baby's cries mean, so I would definitely say put all your energies into feeding her when she cries and then lay her down to sleep again when she's full. It's not as easy to satisfy her with food in that first week, simply because your milk might not have come in enough, and so she'll be hungry, and she'll let you know it! You don't want either of you to be more exhausted in that first week than you need to be, and if your baby won't stop crying because she's hungry it isn't going to be good for either of you.

Crying after the first week ...

It's absolutely pointless me trying to tell you how long your baby may cry in any 24-hour period, as every baby is so different. You might have one who cries for half the day, and you might have one who cries for half an hour.

Chester cried around the clock because he was in pain due to the reflux, but Harry and Belle weren't anywhere near as vocal. Whatever your experience, just go with it and know that nothing lasts forever. With all of mine I found that they were at their worst for crying at between three and six weeks, which is the build-up to their first big developmental milestone at around six weeks – that wonderful first smile!

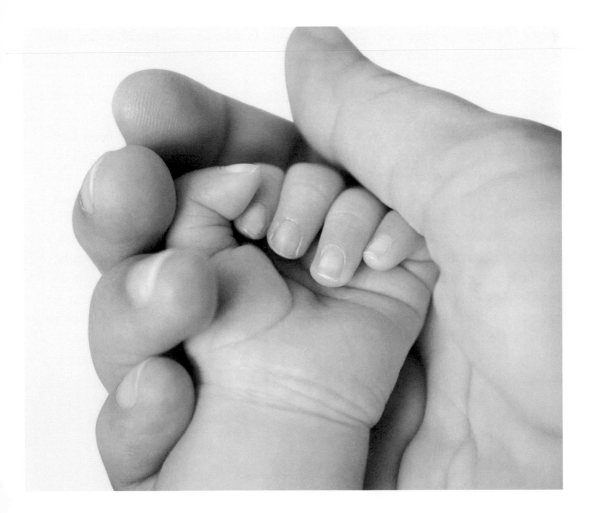

TROUBLESHOOT:
THE CRY BABY

If your baby begins to cry, try to run through this little checklist before you pick up the phone to your GP or health visitor. Babies don't cry for no reason, even if the reason is that they need a cuddle, but if you know that, you know how best to deal with it. They don't always cry because they're in pain either. Every single feeling they are experiencing is a completely new and unknown sensation, so sometimes they just cry because they feel something odd happening, even if it's just feeling a poo coming!

Hungry baby? Is your baby hungry? When was she last fed? Is she going through a growth spurt and in need of more food than last week? There are some widely recognised hungry-baby signs that often accompany a cry, such as rooting towards the breast for food, opening the mouth, and sucking on fingers and hands.

Windy baby? Has your baby been winded enough (see page 43)?

Dirty nappy? Does your baby need a nappy change? Some babies don't care, whilst some hate having a squidgy nappy! So if in doubt, change your baby. I think a wet nappy can make your baby feel cold, so if your baby wakes with a wet nappy in the night after the heating has gone off and you're wondering whether to risk waking her fully to change her, I think it's best to do it. She'll be far more comfortable … in my opinion!

Toilet trouble? Is your baby straining a lot and going red in the face? This can go on for a while until she actually produces a dirty nappy, and can be quite distressing for her. Just offer lots of encouragement, because until she starts to recognise all of her own bodily functions they can all be a little unsettling!

Tired baby? Is your baby tired? Is she getting enough sleep in the daytime (see page 107)?

Poorly baby? Does your baby have a high temperature? Is she teething? Is she bunged up and generally under the weather? If your baby is showing signs of physical pain, give her some infant paracetamol, always following the instructions on the packaging. She can't tell you what's wrong, so you have to read the symptoms and react accordingly.

Too hot or too cold? I've already talked about how babies can't regulate their own body temperatures like older children and adults, so you have to think for them every step of the way. They don't sweat, so don't wait for that sign. The best indicator is to touch a baby's tummy or back of their neck, as their hands and feet aren't an accurate gauge of their temperature.

Lonely baby? Is your baby craving you? She's just spent nearly a year cocooned in the safe environment of your womb, so it's no wonder she craves affection and comfort when she comes out. As I've said before, I don't think you can spoil a baby in the first few months of life, so be on hand with as many cuddles as she needs. She longs for your smell, the sound of your voice and your touch as you shhh, pat and stroke her. Use calming aahs and oohs to soothe her. As long as you balance it out with putting her down on her own to sleep in her Moses basket or cot enough to get her used to it, she'll be fine. Swaddling your baby (see page 123) or putting her in a baby carrier is great for this as she will feel secure, without you having to physically hold her.

Separation anxiety? Up to about six months, babies are fickle little so-and-sos, going to whoever's offering a cuddle, but are you suddenly finding that your baby only wants to come to you? This separation anxiety can happen any time between about six months and a year, and usually comes and goes in waves. The only thing you can do is be there when your baby wants you above anyone else, as she's too young to understand when you tell her you're coming back. Just try to make sure your partner and family are still as involved as they ever were, or you'll end up isolated with your baby. But take heart in the fact that it's just a phase – and get the baby carrier out! It might also be a good time to introduce a favourite soft toy, which will act as a comforter.

SOOTHING TRICKS

Once you've been through the checklist to work out why your baby might be tearful and troubleshooted where you can, try some of these techniques to soothe her, and also take a look at the solution suggestions in the Sleeping chapter, which goes into more detail (see pages 122–132). In the end, you'll develop your own ways to calm your baby, which might be a combination of those below or new methods of your own. Babies respond to different things, so it's a question of trial and error and finding out what works for you.

- Cuddle her close: There is no tonic like a cuddle for a baby. Hold her close – she wants to feel cocooned, warm and secure.

- Talk to her: Nothing is more soothing than the voice she knows and loves.

- Play music or sing to her: Whether she recognises it or not, music can be soothing and have the same effect as white noise. It's all about distraction if you've run through the checklist and tried everything else.

- Shhh/pat/stroke her: Your baby craves your touch, so use it in any way you can to make her feel secure and safe. Imitate the familiar sound of the heartbeat she heard in the womb with your patting rhythm.

- Rock/sway/jiggle her: Your baby has spent the whole time in utero moving with you, so any kind of movement is familiar. Experiment to see what your baby reacts to best.

- Swaddle her or put her in a baby carrier: The same principles about movement apply here, except using a baby carrier leaves you hands-free to get on with your day, and is a godsend if your back is aching from carrying your not-so-tiny, clingy baby around non-stop.

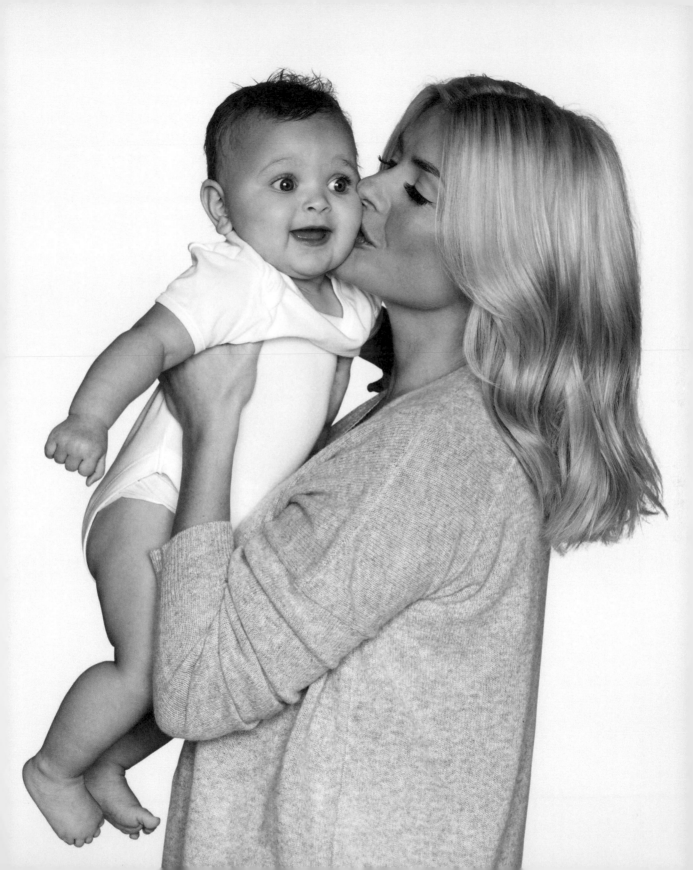

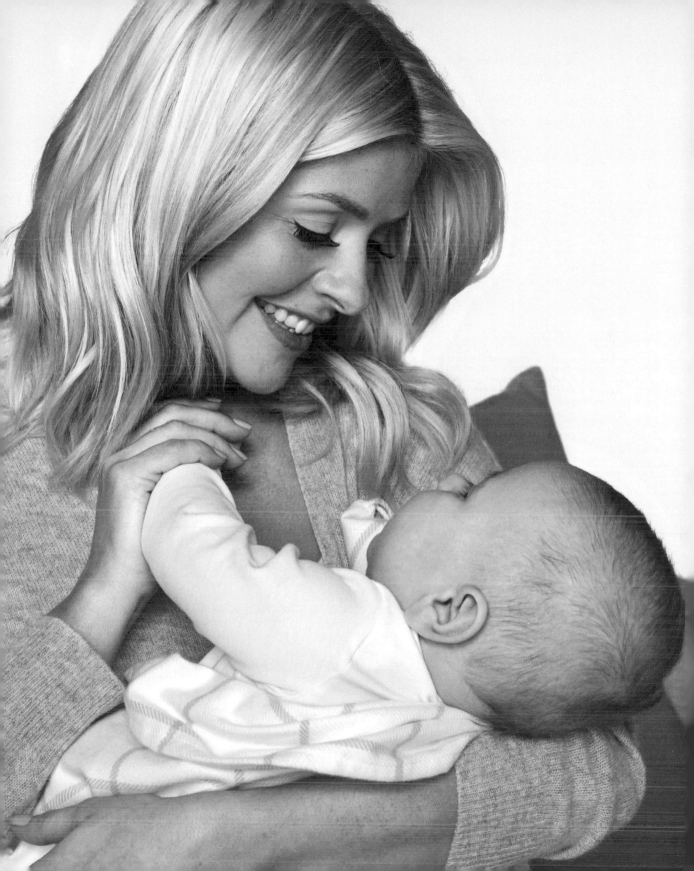

- Use white noise: I've touched on how effective white noise can be to help a baby sleep through other ambient noises around the house (see page 128), but actually I've been known to use it with all of mine during fussy times. Even switching on the hairdryer can break the crying rhythm they've got themselves into, enough to make them forget what they were crying about.

- Have a bath together: The sound of cascading water and the feeling of your skin on her skin in a warm bath can be very soothing to a crying baby. Sometimes it's just the change of scenery that does the trick. Even though you're still in the house, just a change of lighting, taking her clothes off and holding her close can help.

- Give her a dummy or finger to suck: A baby's sucking reflex is very strong, so if you know she's not hungry, just fussing, this might be a good time to give her a dummy or your little finger to suck.

- Go for a walk or a drive: If your baby won't stop crying, wrap her up and get out of the house. A change of scenery and some fresh air will do you the power of good. Go for a drive, even, if you have one of those babies who nods off the second you start the car. It will give you a bit of breathing space, and your baby that longed-for nap. Just be careful not to create a rod for your own back with this or you'll end up driving around all the time to settle her, and bear in mind the safe sleep advice (see page 91). It's better to rock her off for a sleep by taking her for a walk in the pram.

Keep calm Your baby will pick up on your mood, so if you're becoming frustrated and frantic she'll feel it and it will be unnerving. If you are feeling as tired, irritable and frustrated as your crying baby, try doing something to take your mind off it. Try putting on one of your favourite pieces of music – as long as it's calming and not likely to wind her up further!

BABYPROOFING THE HOUSE!

Your home is a potential deathtrap to a baby on the move if you don't take the proper precautions. Like me, you'll want to make sure you've done everything in your power to prevent your little one having an accident. All of these things are simple and inexpensive to do, and could literally save your child's life.

The obvious hazards ...

- Plug sockets: Buy some covers that plug into the holes, taking temptation away from curious little fingers.

- Kitchen and bathroom cupboards: You don't want your baby getting hold of anything poisonous to you, let alone her little body, so invest in some clips or magnets so she can't open cupboard doors containing particularly hazardous products.

- Blinds and curtain cords: Indeed anything that a baby could become tangled in and strangled by. You need to keep everything tightly wound and away from little hands. This is one thing I'm militant about, probably because I met one family on *This Morning* who had fallen victim to losing a child this way. When you sit across from a mother and see the pain in her eyes, there's no going back.

- Stairs: Stairs are an accident waiting to happen, so make sure you have all entrances and exits covered!

- Wires: Keep all wires and cables tucked out of reach to avoid anything being pulled down.

- Kitchen appliances: You need to teach your child as early as possible not to touch hot things, such as hot drinks, and the hob, oven and kettle. Keep all electrical wires tucked safely away.

- Fires: Never leave a child in a room unattended where there's a fire (real or gas), and ensure you have a solid fireguard, one that won't topple onto your baby if she does get close enough.

- Glass-topped tables: Make sure these are made of safety glass. Babies do start to grab and pull themselves up at some point so you don't want them leaning on any surface that isn't toughened. If it's not, you can put a safety cling film over it so if the worst were to happen the broken glass will stay intact.

- Table corners: It's worth buying covers for any sharp corners.

All of that said, babies will eventually need to learn to listen when you say, 'No! Don't touch!' It's all in the tone. A low, stern 'No' should suffice, or a staccato 'Ah … ah … ah!' There's no need to shout, but adjust your tone so that your baby knows you mean business.

If you store away every single breakable or precious item in your house so your baby can't pick it up and smash it, she'll never learn not to touch. Teaching her the concept of 'No' is a crucial part of her development, and when a baby first starts crawling around is a good time to start trying to teach her that there are things she isn't allowed to do or touch.

Out and about …

It goes without saying, but keep an eye on your baby at all times when you take her out of the house! I don't think you can ever be too cautious in this day and age, and equally if your little crawler is in a park or the garden, you want to make sure she's not putting anything in her mouth that she shouldn't be.

If you're taking her out in the car, don't try to multitask. If your baby is crying or needs something, pull over – don't be tempted to solve it on the move. And don't leave your baby unattended in the car. We parents will always worry about people snatching our children, but it's also just dangerous to leave them unattended in case they need you for something, or in case they overheat or get too cold.

03 Growth spurts and developmental milestones

Your baby will grow and change beyond all recognition during her first year of life. You'll watch as that chicken-legged, delicate little squeaker you brought into the world transforms into a confident, happy, squidgy little communicator, who's into absolutely everything she sees!

I can't express enough how important it is to make little notes somewhere about when each of your children did what. Even though you think you'll never forget that your child first sat up at seven months, believe me, once you're a year or so down the road you'll have forgotten everything. It doesn't have to be some meticulously beautiful art project, just a notebook in the kitchen where you can scribble down anything important in between nappy changes! You can also find milestone cards to order online that you can keep to hand so whenever your baby hits one of them you can take a photo of the card next to your baby to mark the date forever!

WHAT YOU CAN EXPECT

There are no set rules when it comes to milestones and development. My children all took their first steps at around a year old, but my niece was toddling at ten months, whilst a friend's daughter didn't walk until 23 months! So don't be discouraged if your baby seems a bit late to join the sitting/crawling/walking party. I've always found that children tend to either be a talker or a walker early on – so you might find you have a really good climber or a really good communicator, and whichever skill she lacks will come later. Childhood is a marathon, not a sprint!

When I met up with my mummy friends we'd find our babies were more challenging in the run-up to a milestone. We'd be moaning about them crying and being clingy, then suddenly they were all sitting up unaided. It's incredible how their little body clocks all work and do what they're supposed to – eventually! One of the most heartbreaking milestones was Harry crying real tears for the first time, at four weeks. It really pulled at the heartstrings!

First month …

Your baby's eyesight is blurry and she has no control at all over her limbs. She is completely reliant on you for anything and everything. That said, she does know your smell and your voice, and she has the grasp reflex for gripping onto your finger and the rooting reflex to find food if you stroke her cheek.

Second month …

This month you might get real tears but also real smiles at around six weeks, which melt your heart. It suddenly becomes clear that your baby is actually smiling at you, as opposed to the usual crooked smile due to some trapped wind. She will begin to see your face more clearly and might even copy some of the movements you make with your mouth if you 'Oooh' and put your tongue out, and she might even gurgle back at you. Your face is the most amazing thing in the world to your baby, so give her as much exposure to it **as possible**.

Third month …

Your baby will be physically much stronger and by the end of this month she will be holding her head aloft and be able to sit face out in the baby carrier. Her eyesight is now perfect, so she can see the toys you've laid out and grab them, rather than just watching whatever it is you're dangling. This is a good time to get her a baby gym mat, so she can have independent play time on her back. Trying to reach up for things is good muscle and movement training.

Fourth month …

This month you might catch your co-ordinated, strong little baby rolling over onto her front! It's much trickier rolling from front to back, so that comes later, but this is a great start. A lovely thing that will happen is that your baby will suddenly notice her hands and they, along with your face, will become the most fascinating things in the world. I can remember all of mine at this point, where they slowly wave their hand in front of their face, following its movement with their eyes. It's too cute – and it keeps them occupied! Double bonus!

◗ Fifth month ...

Now your baby will be experiencing the world via her mouth – putting everything into it – so be aware of what you leave within reach. You'll see her having a look at what she's picked up, then stuffing it into her chops to explore it further. It can also be a sign that there are teeth threatening to make an appearance, but on the whole all babies put everything in their mouths.

◗ Sixth month ...

Your baby might have enough strength and co-ordination to sit up for a few seconds unaided, or roll over from front to back and back to front. Don't panic if yours isn't doing this, though. Just be sure to put down loads of cushions around her, or you can get one of those inflatable doughnut cushions, so that she can sit up supported – whichever way she topples, there's another cushioned edge. It also allows her toys to stay within reach.

It was at this point I made a brilliant purchase – an activity station with a seat. Some of them have seats that rotate and buttons to press that play music. The one I bought wasn't cheap but has literally been loved and coveted by all three of my babies, my nieces and nephews, and some friends' children too! I couldn't recommend it more!

◖ Seventh months to a year ...

If your baby is sitting up and rolling over, she may soon crawl. Some babies move around army-style on their elbows, some bottom-shuffle and some skip crawling altogether! It won't be long before she's pulling herself up to stand, and if you have an early walker she may soon take her first steps! You'll also notice her babbling more than ever, which is adorable (you might even get your first word!). Join in – I actually think babies feel like they're having a conversation, which improves confidence and helps their language to develop.

Developmental fussiness ...

Whilst your baby is exploring her body and the world around her, she will quickly become exhausted and overwhelmed. Deal with this by putting her down for a sleep so she'll be re-energised to have another go when she wakes up. As she develops she might become fussy and irritable through frustration, so bear that in mind when she is unusually over-emotional and clingy.

Everything is still so new and exciting, so it's only natural that your baby might start resisting sleep – yes, the fear of missing out starts that early! You might find her sleeping regresses, which is all to do with how quickly she is developing. She can't tell you how she feels, so she relies on you to help her through it. You just have to make sure you take charge and ensure she's getting enough sleep and rest, or all of your wheels will fall off!

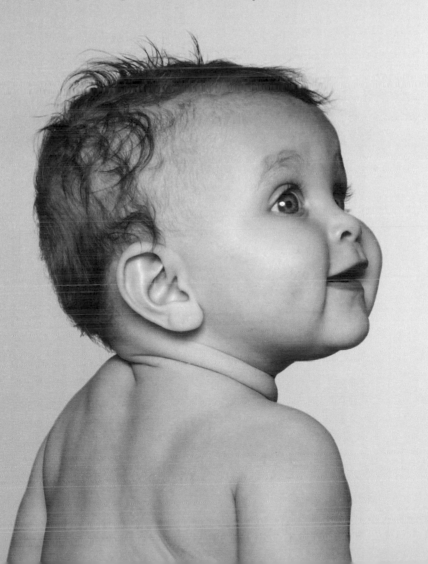

Summary Hopefully that little lot will help allay some of your fears and guide you through the first year. Most of it really is common sense and I'm sure you'll do just great. You know best how to care for your baby – just listen to that know-it-all intuition of yours and you won't go wrong.

If in doubt, always seek advice from fellow mums, your family and friends, or, if it concerns your child's health, a medical professional.

WELLBEING

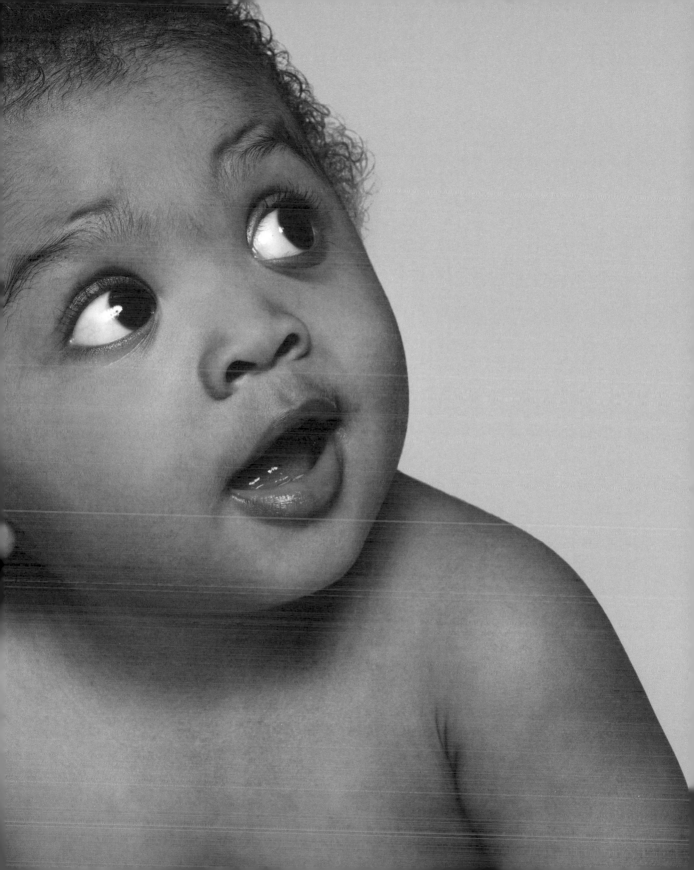

Lifestyle

- CHAPTER FOUR -

How much will my life change now I have a baby?

You won't be surprised to hear that it'll change quite a bit! You will have already made some inroads during pregnancy, but when your baby arrives the shift will be complete. Be reassured that this change happens in phases, which will alter again as your baby grows and his needs evolve, so nothing is permanent or for very long. You won't always be tied to your own front room, as you are in those first couple of months. It's just until you feel ready to venture out and are comfortable enough to trust a babysitter. Remember, just because your life is different, it doesn't mean you are. You're the same person, it's just that now you have a permanent plus-one to consider, who's the new centre of your life.

So this chapter is all about the things you'll find yourself thinking about now you're a mum – from affording your new addition and what you'll do with your days with a baby in tow, to giving your baby a fulfilling and fun little lifestyle of his own!

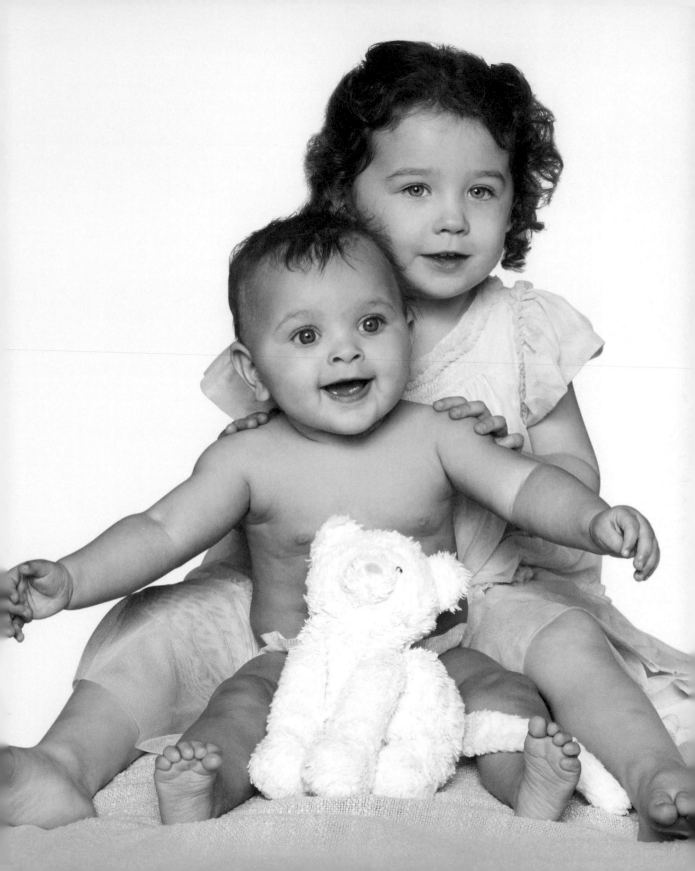

01 The serious stuff

Now this is where I talk to you about all the important little admin bits for you and your new little person – everything from registering your baby to thinking about family cars.

I've also tried to give some tips on affording a baby, which can be pretty daunting at first – but you'll hopefully find that staying in is definitely the new going out, whether it's just sitting in with your partner and ordering a takeaway, or going to a friend's house with your baby and putting him down to sleep there, whilst you let your hair down for the evening. You'll suddenly start having sleepovers again if your friends have the room! It's hilarious!

OFFICIAL BUSINESS TO REMEMBER

Registering your baby …

I'm including the registration of your baby here because those first few weeks can whizz by and before you know it the deadline for registering your child as an official person is upon you. By law, you have to register your child within 42 days of the birth at your local register office (see page 281). If you're married to the father of your baby, either you or your spouse can register the birth. If you aren't, but want both of your names to appear on the birth certificate, you will have to attend the appointment together.

You will both need to take a form of identification, as well as your baby's little red PCHR book (see page 155), and have decided on your baby's name(s). I would recommend paying for an extra copy or two of your baby's birth certificate rather than having to apply for duplicates further down the road. It's always a worry when you have to post off a copy of the certificate to apply for a passport, for example, so knowing that you've got a spare original at home will definitely give you peace of mind.

Passport application …

Once you've registered your baby you can apply for a passport for him, if you're planning to go abroad in the not too distant future. Children's passports only last for five years, though, so it's a good idea to put a reminder in your diary to apply for a new one at least six months before it expires (most countries require six months' validity on a passport before granting entry). I've actually done that with all my family's passports because I'm worried I'll only notice it's nearly expired when I'm on the way to the airport!

211

LIFESTYLE

AFFORDING A BABY

Watch what you buy ...

There's no denying it, an extra person in your life is going to push your monthly outgoings up. By how much will depend on how clever and resourceful you are, so think carefully before loading up your credit card. There are some ridiculous lists of baby 'must-haves', but don't be drawn in. You don't need every single thing on the baby market. It's natural for you to want your new baby to have the best, but not everything has to be brand new! Babies grow out of things quickly, so assess whether it's worth the money. Of course there will be some things that from a health and safety perspective you want to buy new, such as a mattress for your second-hand cot, teats for bottles, and dummies. Don't feel pressured to furnish your nursery with everything all at once. There's plenty of time to pick up the things you really need as you go along, and you'll need an excuse to get out of the house and to the shops!

Ask for advice ...

Another thing I did, after studying that 100-page-long internet list of what you need to buy, was ask all my mummy friends for one thing they couldn't have done without and one thing they wished they'd never wasted their money on, then I stocked up accordingly. They all said the fewer things you have cluttering up the kitchen work surface, the better – so, for example, don't buy a bottle warmer when standing a bottle in a bowl of hot water will do! Many said they couldn't live without a baby carrier – to leave you hands-free carrying your little fusspot around the house, rescuing your aching back in the process.

FOC (free of charge, mummy!) ...

It's worth asking those friends and family who've had children if they've got any equipment knocking about that their children have outgrown. You'll be surprised how many things you'll amass FOC! We've got things that have been passed around lots by family and friends. It's lovely to have something that's done the rounds and comes back to you for your next child. Invest in some baby-friendly antibacterial spray to clean everything. If you're lending baby clothes, only offer those things you'll be happy not to get back and not anything you love and want to keep for other children in the future. Nine times out of ten, your bright whites will come back grey!

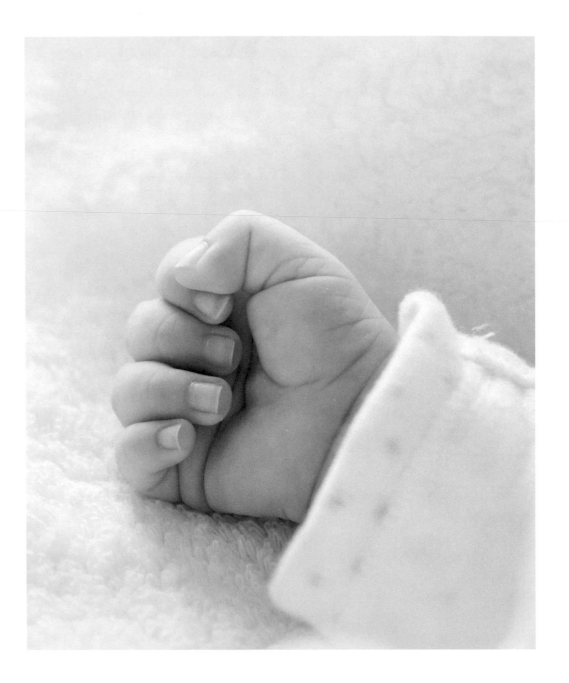

Charity shops ...

These can be brilliant, particularly the specialist children's ones. I'm sure you're probably reading this and thinking 'Really? Holly shops in charity shops?' But I really do! I've got a wonderful children's charity shop just up the road from me and I don't think I've ever walked past it without having a glance in the window or going in. So try it! Mark my words, one day that pink bouncer you've been hankering after will appear for all of £3! Charity shops are great for those things children lose every five minutes, like gloves and hats. The cheeky little so-and-sos whip them off so fast and fling them out of the pram, and you don't even notice they're gone until you get home. There's absolutely no point in spending on things like that and charity shops usually have baskets full of them. You might even find the glove you're missing! They should also be your first port of call if you've gone for a walk and suddenly found yourself in the middle of an unpredicted rainstorm, to nip in and pick up an umbrella or hat for you!

Financial support ...

Your child might be eligible for a weekly child benefit allowance up to the age of 16 depending on your income, but you have to apply for it as soon as you have registered your baby and provide a birth certificate to accompany the application. The money is paid into one parent's account, and there might be other tax credits and things you can apply for, depending on your financial status, so make sure you go to the government portal to find out exactly what you and your family are entitled to (see page 281).

A word to the wise ...

Hopefully things will balance up enough for you to get through this costly time because you'll probably be spending less in other areas. For example, you may no longer be going out for a drink or to eat once a week whilst you settle into life with your new baby, so the money you would have spent on social events will be there to pay for nappies. Don't get depressed by this thought! It won't be forever! And you'll find your social life will probably move from the pub to eating in at some other parent's house anyway.

The main thing is to work out a budget and do your best to stick to it. Make sure you and your partner communicate any money worries, so that you can work on the best plan of action together. Internalising things like financial difficulties at a time when you're exhausted and at your most vulnerable is just going to make you miserable and in the wrong state of mind as a new mother with an extremely dependent baby to care for.

TRAVEL

Car seats and pram systems ...

There are so many pram systems on the market now – the only thing you can do is physically go out and test drive as many as you can. My priorities when selecting ours were to have a car seat that fitted straight onto the pram without having to add any attachments, and a pram that folded up super-easily. You'll be surprised at how many times a day you end up folding and unfolding your pram, so to have one that requires the minimum amount of effort and fuss is crucial! Last, for me, was good manoeuvrability. I never got on very well with a two-handled pram as you can't steer it one handed whilst attending to your child with the other. I chose a pram with one handlebar that was easy to push around corners. You'll be permanently pushing that pram for the first year so, if you can, invest in one that does most of the work!

Buying a family car ...

Ask yourself how many children you want to have. I always knew I wanted three, so when it was our time to look for a family car I did my research and chose a car that would comfortably fit three car seats/booster seats in a row. I looked for one that was economical to run and where you could use all the seats, fit in a grandparent or one of the children's friends and still fit a pram in the boot. This might sound crazy, but these are all important questions you should be asking yourself before you make such a big investment!

I also think whilst you have a young family your car is going to have, at best, a rice cake squished into the upholstery, or at worst get pooped on. So know that these messy times are coming, and relax. But maybe this is easy for me to say as someone who isn't really a car person! Hey, sports cars are for your mid-life crisis, right? Now you know why!

02 Development and play

All the way through your child's development, your face, your voice, your touch and your smell will provide the most interesting and comforting stimulation. Babies will find anything fascinating and, more often than not, their favourite thing won't be a toy at all, but your face, or your keys, which of course aren't at all sterile! You acting the clown, pulling faces, blowing raspberries and doing silly voices will be more entertaining than any toy.

Having said that, there's a lot to be said for having one or two good baby toys up your sleeve to entertain your baby with when what he really needs is a change of scenery, but you're stuck in a waiting room … waiting!

TOYS

You absolutely do not need to spend a fortune at the nearest toy shop! Of course you'll accrue some new toys, whether it's because you just couldn't help yourself or they are gifts from other people. If you do want to buy toys, why not look in your local children's charity shop? As long as you give everything a good wipe down with some baby-friendly antibacterial spray when you get it home to sterilise it, whether it's for a three-month-old or a five-year-old, they'll never know the difference and you'll have more money in your pocket to put towards a weekend activity!

The MOST important thing to check, particularly in your baby's first year, when your baby is exploring absolutely everything with his mouth, is to make sure all toys are age-appropriate, and if they're handmade that you're 100 per cent confident they're completely sealed.

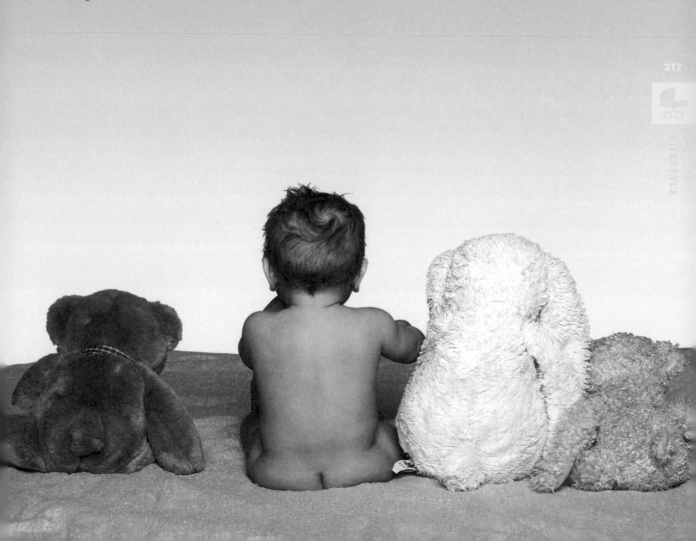

Early toys ...

Babies react well to black-and-white images and vibrant colours, so if you've filled the nursery with beautiful pure white, then get some primary colours in your life! The louder the colours and the more things dangling, the better. Many come with an attachment ring to secure them to the pram or car seat and stop you losing them when you're out and about. Any toy with a mirror is always good, as babies are as fascinated with their own reflection as they are with your face.

As babies grow and want more independence, you might want to invest in a play mat – but, again, check out charity shops before you pay full price. As your baby's eyesight and co-ordination improve, he'll want things he can aim for and grab at. Mobiles that move are also great at this stage, as are books with different textures, flaps and noise buttons. Babies love anything that rattles or crunches as they grab it.

Homemade toys for all ages ...

Things you've made at home can be just as thrilling as shop-bought toys – just make sure they're completely safe and age-appropriate. All you need is a sealable, non-breakable container and something noisy to put in it – for example, pasta shapes in a plastic water bottle make a lovely rattle, or you can simply put water in a bottle for your baby to shake – he'll love watching it move. As your baby gets older, you can add food colouring or glitter to the contents. Kitchen utensils such as wooden spoons, measuring spoons, silicone whisks and a spatula always seem to be firm favourites, as children feel like they're playing with grown-up toys! Just make sure you keep everything clean.

Washing toys My children always managed to throw up on toys, so any that could go through the washing machine did. Be careful with bath toys. Those squeezy ones quite often collect mould inside, so if they look a bit dark throw them out or put them through the dishwasher – you don't want your baby chewing them and swallowing anything nasty.

INTERACTION & MOVEMENT

Games ...

There are plenty of games you can play without needing any props, from tickling your baby to whooshing him up in the air, to repeating nursery rhymes such as 'This Little Piggy' with accompanying actions. Games like peekaboo are lifelong favourites, and both fun and educational for your baby. You might wonder why he never seems to tire of the game. I mean, really, how funny can it be?! Once he knows your face will reappear, surely it will get boring after 20 or so times. But because babies don't have object permanence, when you hide your face and then reappear, they're surprised and excited because they'd quite forgotten you were there in the first place!

Once your baby gets to grips with object permanence, playing peekaboo becomes a good way to teach him that just because he can't see you, you haven't gone forever and you will come back. This is great for helping with separation anxiety.

Sing or play music …

Singing nursery rhymes and songs over and over again is a great way for your baby to absorb language and vocabulary without even realising it. Try 'Round and Round the Garden', 'The Wheels on the Bus', 'Wind the Bobbin Up', 'I'm a Little Teapot', 'Incy Wincy Spider' and 'Zoom, Zoom, Zoom', and if you're feeling really brave, throw in some actions! I'm sure the internet is full of nursery rhyme dance routines!

Have a conversation …

Babies babble and coo, and you can literally while away hours watching over them on their play mat. If there's a break in your baby's babble, use it as your cue to answer him with similar sounds – you might find he answers you back. There you have it … your first conversation. It's adorable, and even though it's utter gobbledygook you'll both get a kick out of it.

Talk to him and show him things …

As your baby grows, talk to him properly, not just using baby language. Explain things using the proper terminology and read picture books to him, especially ones that rhyme (eventually they will help prompt your baby on the word that will come next). You never know what's going into those pulsating memory banks of his. The repetitive use of language over and over again becomes familiar and, eventually, he'll repeat it back to you. Think how many songs you know the words to and have no idea when you learnt them. It's just from hearing them over and over again on the radio! Eventually they go in subconsciously.

Make sure to point things out to him wherever you are. You may feel like a mad woman talking and joking with your baby as you walk around the supermarket, but that's honestly the best sort of stimulation for him and how he will learn. Children's minds are like sponges, and even though you think your baby has no idea what it is you're saying to him – which he probably doesn't – it won't be long before he starts reacting appropriately. You'll get the shock of your life when you ask him where his toes are and he looks down and grabs them. He was listening after all! I can remember one time driving along on a very rare occasion without any children in the back and becoming aware I was muttering, 'Car … car … bus … fire engine … car … bike … car,' under my breath. I'd been so used to pointing out every single moving vehicle to Harry, it was now second nature! See … you do become a crazy woman!

Baby signing …

I have to say that I didn't do baby signing with any of my children – not for any reason other than I didn't have the opportunity to, with everything else that was going on. I had a friend who was a big advocate of it and the results were quite extraordinary for a baby so young. We know that babies are like sponges, in particular in the way they mimic behaviour and movements, so baby signing is a way of capitalising on that to teach them how to express what they want or need through gestures before their language has developed.

There is a school of thought that says if you give a child the option of communicating in a way other than verbally, the child may continue to rely on that, rather than progressing with proper speech. But I'm assured that's not the way it works. Because you're speaking the words at the same time as doing the actions, the idea is that your baby is absorbing vocabulary too. I think anything that involves you interacting with your baby is key to language development, so if this puts an interesting spin on things for you, then do your own research and go for it!

Give your baby space to explore …

As babies grow, they don't always want to be held or hovered over! It's good for them to have a kick-about on a play mat. Or if it's summer time, take your baby to the park and lay him on a rug (in the shade). Whether he's at lying, sitting, crawling or toddling stage, it's important not to hover over him. Of course, I hear myself say this and think, of course you should watch his every move, but I mean give him space to figure things out for himself. If you're always there to hold him up or catch him, he'll never learn to do it alone. Give him as much independence as you can in the safest environment possible so no real harm can come to him, and watch him grow in confidence.

Tummy time ...

Your midwife and health visitor will tell you the crucial attributes of tummy time, which is literally placing your baby on his tummy for small intervals and watching as he tries to lift his head clear. The main reason it's recommended is because babies are now put down to sleep on their back so spend very little time on their tummy, and it's supposedly the only way your baby's muscles will develop enough to support his back and neck. I can see why this is important, but can honestly say not all my children took to it.

I think with everything, as long as you're giving it a go and giving your baby the opportunity to experience everything he should, then you're doing enough. Some babies just hate being on their front. They might get used to it if you leave them on their tummy a little bit more every time, but they might not. Unless there's something medically wrong, most children can sit up and roll over by the time they are aged one, so they'll get there eventually.

PRESERVING THE MEMORIES

Photos and videos …

We are lucky enough to live in a digital age where the ability to photograph and video is literally at our fingertips – our mobiles! Just make sure you remember to download any footage you take in case you drop your phone down the toilet when you're multitasking five thousand things (as usual!).

Email account …

I have to admit I've never done it, but someone told me about setting up an email account for your child and emailing notes, images and videos whenever you think about it, as a kind of life diary – and then giving your child the address and password on his 18th birthday or when he's old enough to appreciate it. This is such an adorable idea, but of course it will take time and dedication.

Memory box …

Get yourself a memory box so you can keep all your little baby-related trinkets together. It doesn't have to be anything fancier than a shoebox, but it will be lovely to keep and for you to go through with your spotty teenager one day! I've got baby boxes for all of mine, crammed with the lock of hair from their first haircut, my favourite babygro, and all their first birthday and Christmas cards, etc. Perhaps I'm hoarding a bit too much, but I can't help it!

There are plenty of other creative things you can do to capture your baby in time. Going to a pottery café where you'll make plates and mugs with your child's foot and handprints on is a lovely thing to do – and these make great presents for grandparents! You can buy DIY clay or plaster impression kits where you mould your child's feet and hands. There are companies that make bronze sculptures for you or take fingerprint impressions and make keyrings or cufflinks from them. You can send your favourite items of clothing or muslins off and they get sent back as a quilt or as art for the wall. Shall I go on?!

The first birthday party ...

You'll hum and haw about what to do for the all-important first-ever birthday! Whether you go all out and have ponies dressed as unicorns and clowns on stilts, or get together with a couple of other mums whose babies were born around the same time and have a shared tea party, one thing's for sure – as long as you get that all-important photo of your baby wearing a token party hat in front of a cake with one lit candle, you'll have done your bit!

One great thing I must share, which I think started in the US, is to make your baby a separate cake, smother it in soft butter icing, place it in the middle of some plastic sheeting, strip your baby down to his nappy and let him crawl over and demolish it at will. From the photos I've seen, it looks amazing and such fun!

03 What to do with your days

If you worked full-time, you might find it tricky adapting to life at home with just your baby for company (wonderful as he is!). But unless you live up a mountain in the Himalayas, the odds are you'll find plenty of local mother and baby groups so, when you feel ready, try out a few. Check your GP's surgery noticeboard, your local pharmacy, or have a look at mummy-specific websites (see page 281) to find out what's available.

These groups are a great way to get out of the house and pass a few hours, and they will provide stimulation for your baby and exposure to other babies. Most importantly, they are a way to meet other like-minded, exhausted mummies! The majority take place in churches, civic halls or children's centres, and there's usually a friendly face to greet you with a cup of tea. Not every class will break the bank either, costing just a couple of pounds for a session – well worth it if only for the change of scenery! I've also covered things to think about if you want to take your baby on holiday. Piña colada, anyone?!

Postnatal groups …

If you met mums at antenatal classes, it might be worth meeting up with them now. Your babies will have been born within days or weeks of each other, so the chances are you'll all be going through the same thing at the same time. There's no better tonic than talking through problems with like-minded people and swapping survival tips. I was lucky enough to make a couple of good friends in my antenatal classes, but if you don't get so lucky (it's complete luck of the draw), look for other ways to meet new mums.

Baby sing-along and music groups …

I've taken all of mine to a local weekly baby sing-along group. You'll be amazed how quickly babies seem to recognise songs like 'Incy Wincy Spider'. It can be good exercise too, as you lift your little one up and down to the music! Drop-in, pay-as-you-go groups are probably a better idea in the early days as you never know when you're going to have a particularly bad night and be too exhausted to leave the house. There's nothing good about feeling pressured to go to something just because you've already paid for it. There might also be the option to buy a book of ten sessions, to be used up over twelve months, for example. Just arrive early to avoid disappointment, then once you find something you're confident your baby enjoys, it can be cheaper to sign up to a term of classes.

Be prepared Keep a ready-stocked changing bag by the front door, complete with nappies, wet wipes, nappy cream, nappy bags, a spare change of clothes, bibs, sterilised dummies, etc. The only things you'll need to add before you leave are formula, snacks and bottles.

Baby massage and baby yoga ...

Both these activities use touch and movement to stimulate a baby's senses. Your baby spends most of the time on his back or strapped in a car seat, so you can see why massage and yoga would benefit him. You are moving and stimulating parts of your baby's body that might otherwise remain quite still.

Most places suggest baby massage from about four to six weeks old, whilst baby yoga tends to start at around three months. The massage class is more a learning curve for you, where you are taught how to massage your baby for relaxation at home. Your baby will enjoy it during the class, but massage is best done after bathtime as a quiet and relaxing activity before bed (see page 116, and also pages 186-7 for a few ideas). These classes are a lovely way for you to spend a few hours together and with other new mummies.

Baby swimming ...

I took all of my children to baby swimming classes from three months after they'd had their first injections. By three months, most babies love being in the water, and it's an added bonus for your baby to be held close to one of his favourite people ... you! It's also a great idea to get him used to being in the water, and even under it, to set him on the path to becoming a confident swimmer later in life.

Whether you attend a course or take your baby to the local pool, you'll probably have to put him in a swimming nappy covered by a special neoprene, leak-free nappy cover, which protects the water and everyone else in it from any unwanted, unexpected nasties! I would advise against a swim session if your baby has a cold, as he will chill off quickly in the water, particularly when he's really young. Also, if you have a baby with sensitive skin, or any eczema-type skin conditions, the chlorine can aggravate these. Always rinse the chlorine off your baby after swimming. You can buy neoprene baby wetsuits as an extra layer of warmth for young babies whilst swimming. They also protect against direct sunlight in hot weather, but make sure your baby doesn't overheat.

At the end of your first term, some swimming clubs offer the opportunity to get an underwater photo with your baby, and I have to say that these are some of my most favourite photos I've got of the kids. They remind me of the Nirvana *Nevermind* album cover!

Buggy fitness …

Once you've had your six-week check and been given the all-clear to exercise, it's never too early for your baby to be exposed to a healthy fitness regime – even if he is just spectating as you sweat!

Buggy fitness can be as simple as taking your baby for a walk, but if you want to combine getting fit with meeting like-minded mums and harnessing the power of the group workout, there are plenty of buggy fitness groups up and down the country. The good thing about these groups is that you take your baby with you in the buggy, which is great as it means you don't have to organise childcare, and he can stay with you and at the same time get plenty of fresh air. The fact that you're pushing a buggy gives your body an all-over workout, because you're not just using your legs as you walk or jog, but your arms and core too as you steer the buggy.

You don't have to go to a specific class for this, though. When I was on maternity leave with Chester, I used to walk Harry and Belle to school with Chester in the buggy, and then a couple of the other mums – some with babies, some not – would join me for a brisk walk after drop-off.

Baby-friendly cinema ...

Cinemas up and down the country offer special baby-friendly screenings for mothers and babies. It's a completely calm and lovely experience, and one where you don't need to worry if your child has a meltdown. Every other audience member in the auditorium will be praying their baby won't be the next to kick off!

I have to say, though, that something about the sound and the darkness – even though the sound has been turned down and the lighting increased from your usual grown-up cinema experience – seems to subdue and calm the babies, and they nod off to sleep immediately, leaving you to watch the film or catch a few zzzs yourself. It's usually a grown-up movie, too, so something that will appeal to you.

Children's story time ...

My local pub used to do story time once a week for babies and toddlers. It was great as it was literally up the road, and another opportunity to get out of the house and connect with local mums. You can also check your local library for these sorts of sessions.

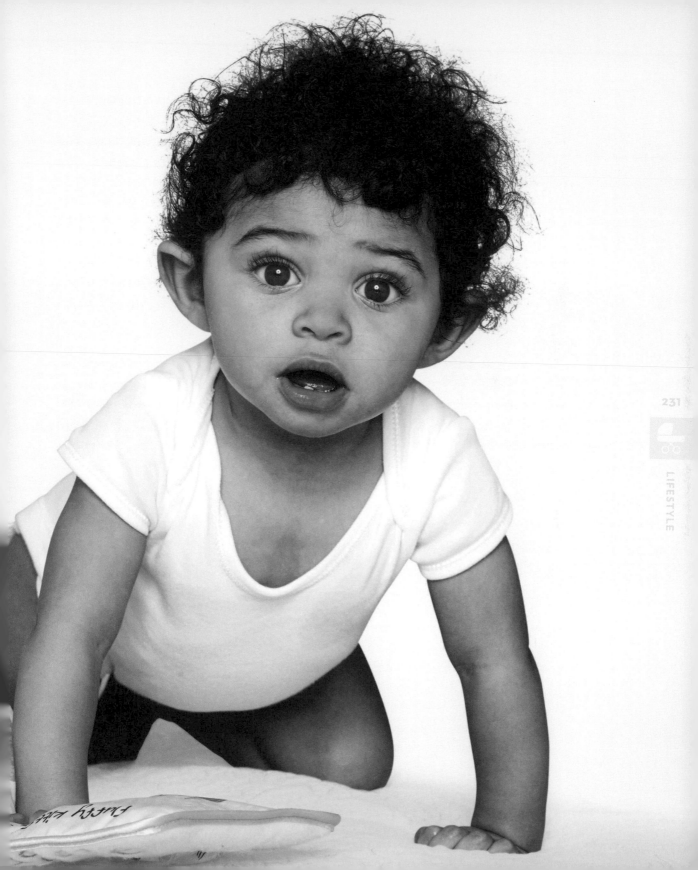

ADAPTING TO LIFE AS A
STAY-AT-HOME MUM

If you've always been used to working a full-time job, maternity leave can fluctuate between being wonderful and, at times, a bit of a struggle. You might feel like your brain has turned to mush and wonder if you'll ever be the bright-spark career woman again. There might be mornings you wish you were off to do the morning commute and your partner was going to walk a day in your shoes, just for a bit of adult company and a taster of your old life as a girl about town! There's nothing wrong with having these feelings – they're completely natural. You've spent so much of your life as an independent woman, it would be odd if you didn't miss it sometimes. And it doesn't make you a bad mum, it might just mean you need a break, or that you need to try not to be so isolated.

The more things you do with your baby in the day and the more contact you have with other mums, the quicker the days will pass and the easier it will be. It might not be long before you're back in the rat race, so try to adapt and enjoy the moment. After the first month or so, maternity leave goes by in a flash, and probably comes to an end just when you start getting used to it!

Things you can do to stay sane ...

If your baby's sleeping, don't automatically pick up the washing basket or peel some potatoes. If you're caring for your baby and doing chores around the clock, with no YOU time, you'll go crazy!

- **Get some sleep:** Sleep when your baby sleeps. You need it!

- **Eat a proper meal:** Even if it's beans on toast and a cup of tea, and don't move until you've finished both whilst they're still hot!

- **Wash and blow-dry your hair:** Step away from the dry shampoo! Sometimes it's the smallest things that become a missed luxury after you've had a baby. Things you took for granted in your 'single' life that can make you feel a million times better.

- **Online shopping:** Even if it's only window shopping and you don't actually order anything, online shopping can make you feel in touch with the outside world in the early days. Don't get into the rut of only ever ordering a supermarket shop; occasionally it's OK to order yourself a treat.

- **Pick up the phone:** Have a chat to a friend about anything – even better, a friend without children so you can have a non-baby-related discussion for ten minutes and feel less alienated.

- **Read something adult:** And by that I don't mean something X-rated! I mean pick up a book or a newspaper, or read a magazine online – something that stimulates your mind and reminds you that you did once have a brain that you used beyond working out the hours between feeds!

- **Do some exercise:** Even if it's a walk around the block for ten minutes all by yourself whilst your mum or someone else listens out for the baby.

However you feel your life has changed after having a baby, just know that babies are as adaptable as you make them and can fit in with pretty much anything as long as they're getting the food, sleep and love they need. Take me, for example. Five weeks after having Harry I went for my six-week check with my GP on the way to the *X Factor* holding room for auditions! I was hosting *The Xtra Factor* at the time and had to be there, so I took Harry and my mum with me and breastfed him around filming.

 Thinking back, it was a bit crazy and I don't know how it worked, but thanks to Harry being such a good feeder and my mum being there, it just did! I can remember that holding room now, full of families supporting contestants who might be sitting there from 9am to 9pm waiting to audition – families with babies, and every time I heard a baby cry my boobs would fill up with milk and I'd have to rush to the toilet to change my breast pad, or feed Harry! Not a particularly conducive environment for a new mum, but a good example of how flexible you and your baby can be.

HOLIDAYS

Spending time together as a family on holiday can produce some of your most magical memories so, if you have the opportunity, I would definitely recommend it. Travelling abroad with a baby can be daunting but, as with everything, if you're organised you'll be fine. You don't have to pay for an airline seat for your baby until his second birthday, so if you're lucky enough to be in the financial position to do so, go on holiday as often as you can!

If you are flying long haul, don't worry about the time difference or how to get a baby back on track; you can do this when you get home in a few days. In fact, you can easily get babies back into a routine by adjusting their day sleeps.

Your destination …

If you're going somewhere hot, keep your baby in the shade as much as possible, and when he is in the water a UV bodysuit is best to protect his sensitive skin. You'll need a high-factor, specially formulated sun cream for babies (check the age range) and a hat he can't pull off. You can also buy baby sunglasses with elastic that goes around the head. A buggy shade is a good idea, so you can protect your baby from the sun whilst he is asleep in the pram during the day.

Check what baby facilities are available at your hotel. You don't want to come unstuck and arrive somewhere where there isn't a cot or a kettle to heat water for a bottle. Most hotels are family-friendly, though, so should have everything you need. I wouldn't worry about taking your own cot bedding as cots come in all shapes and sizes, so you'll never get it right. If there isn't a clean fitted sheet, use one of the spare bed sheets and fold it over to the mattress size. But always make sure it's tucked tightly under the mattress so it can't work its way out and become a suffocation risk. Put your baby in his baby sleeping bag on top, which you know is clean and familiar to him, so hopefully you'll all get a good night's sleep!

Depending on the type of accommodation, you may or may not have a bottle steriliser available. It's a good idea to take sterilising tablets with you, though, so that you can clean a bottle or dummy wherever there's water!

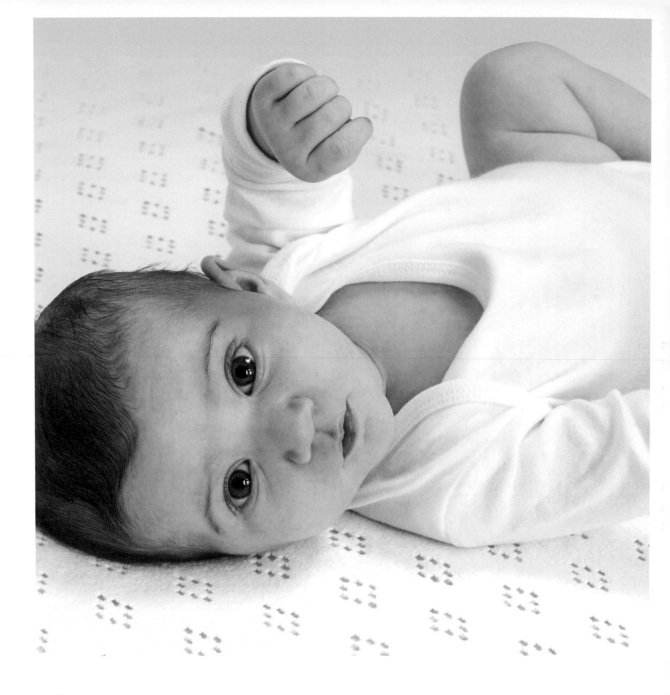

Night flights If possible, take a night flight so that it fits in with your baby's natural sleeping pattern as he's much more likely to go off for the whole flight.

Luggage allowance ...

Most airlines allow you two items of extra check-in luggage – choose from a buggy, travel cot or car seat. If you take a car seat, get a car-seat bag – you can pack nappies and wet wipes inside to lighten your luggage load. When you're on board you'll be allocated a bulkhead where your baby can sleep in an airline cot instead of him being on your lap, but these are first come, first served, so try to book ahead or check in early to avoid disappointment.

How to get through the flight ...

It's a good idea to pack a couple of toys your baby hasn't seen before so he has something new to entertain him during the flight. If you have an older child, you could even wrap these toys up like presents to add to the novelty! But, in all honesty, the chances are it will be the rustling crisp packet, not the toys, that keeps your baby entertained! I think that if you go onto a flight with an open mind and an open heart, knowing that at worst you'll spend the entire time walking up and down the plane with your baby, then you'll be fine.

In-flight food ...

If you're not breastfeeding, take plenty of sterilised bottles in your hand luggage and you can buy the ready-made formula cartons airside. I phoned and reserved some once as I was in a panic they might be sold out, but they always have plenty. You can take bottles of cooled boiled water, but you will be asked to taste one of them at security to check it is what you're saying it is.

Take-off and landing Feed your baby during take-off and landing as it will equalise the pressure in his ears. If your baby has a dummy, sucking that has the same effect.

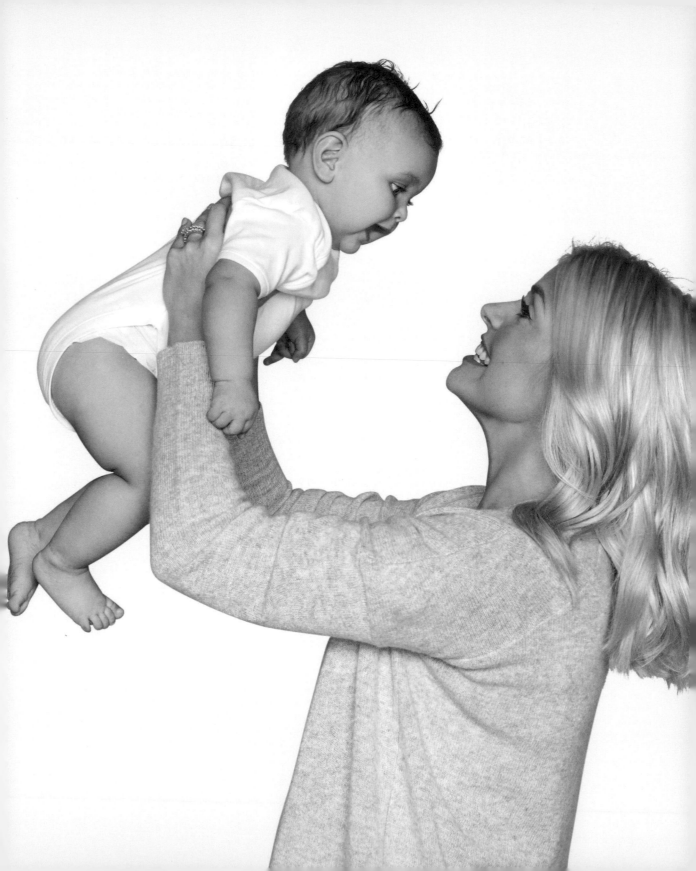

Summary So there you have it, mummy – lots of ideas to keep you and your bundle busy!

The most encouraging day you can have is one spent with other mums who are experiencing the same highs and lows. So why not try a baby class and capitalise on all those lovely endorphins you get from doing a bit of exercise? It doesn't have to be anything strenuous, just try to get moving a bit!

Try not to put too much of a financial strain on yourselves. Your baby will never know or care if his toys were brand new or much-loved and played-with hand-me-downs. Your baby will grow to be a wonderful human being not because of what he had, but because you were there to love and guide him. And that really is all that matters.

Be there for your baby, love your baby, and the life you lead as a family will be the envy of everyone lucky enough to be part of it.

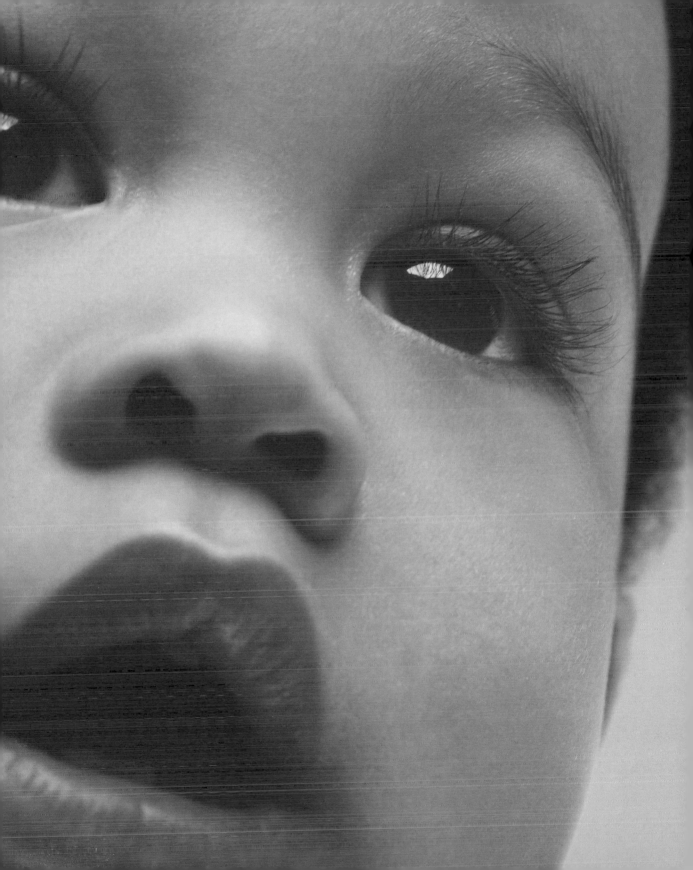

Looking after you

- CHAPTER FIVE -

✻

I love my new baby, but will I ever feel like me again?!

Yes, do not despair! There are likely to be times when you look at yourself in the mirror and think, 'Is this really who I am now?' Most new mums have gone through these moments. Hang on in there! Unless you're very lucky or Superwoman, you're probably sleep-deprived and still in possession of your post-baby jelly-belly, and so feeling a bit low and fed up. These thoughts don't make you a bad mother or ungrateful for your baby. Instead, try looking in the mirror and thinking, 'YES! This is who I am now. I'm amazing! I've just given birth to the most precious thing in the world.'

In this chapter I'll talk about some of the things you might be experiencing, both emotionally and physically, in your new life as a yummy mummy. The most important thing to remember is to take note of how you are feeling and seek help if there are any odd changes. It's so easy to disregard yourself when your baby arrives because she needs so much from you, but it's really important that *you* stay healthy and well, or the wheels will fall off!

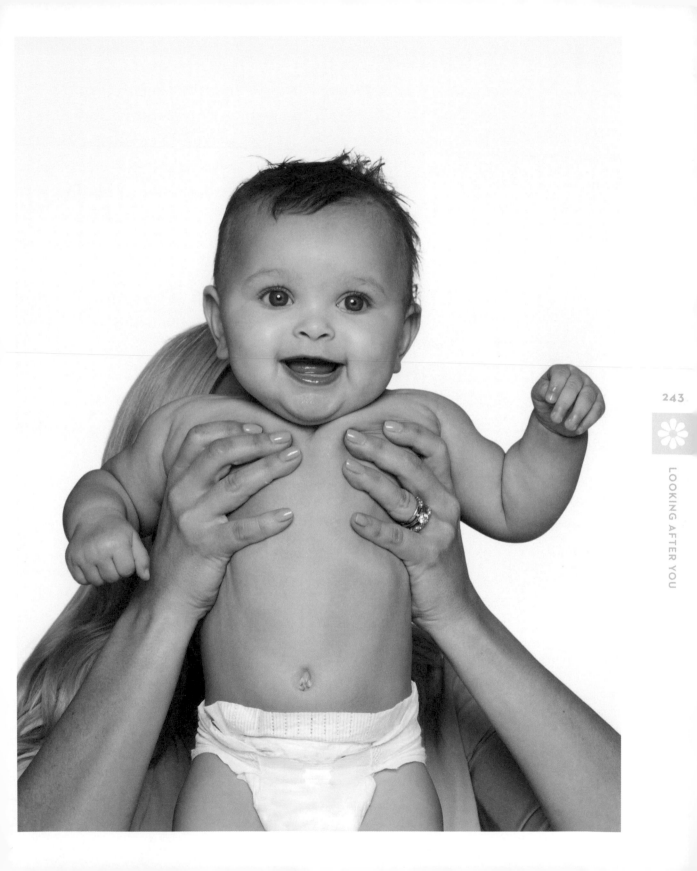

01 What's going on with you?!

Pregnancy and giving birth really take their toll on your body, so don't expect everything to ping back to normal straight away. In this section I've tried to prepare you for what to expect physically, and offer advice on how to deal with any discomfort and pain.

As well as the physical changes, be prepared for a bit of an emotional rollercoaster too. After the high of giving birth – the relief your baby is here and the amazement of meeting her – you may hit a low. This is completely normal. Like some women, you may not be completely in love with your baby just yet, and processing that emotion can be hard.

To be honest, the weeks after having a baby can be a complete minefield. You're tired and your hormones are all over the place, so be patient and cut yourself some slack. Any negatives are temporary and, believe me, you have positives ahead. Just remember that, whatever your thoughts or feelings, you are not alone. The new mother in the next street is probably feeling exactly the same thing, as your lives mirror each other – lights flicking on and off through the night as you're both up feeding your hungry babies!

POSTNATAL FACTS OF LIFE

Everything aches ...

Giving birth puts a massive strain on your body and you'll discover aches and pains in muscles you never knew existed! Think about it this way – you might have been in labour for a couple of days, meaning your body was under constant strain for hours on end. Anything else resulting in that kind of impact and you'd have been in training for weeks, so is it any wonder that you ache from head to toe?! It will get better, though, just in the same way that aches and pains go away after any vigorous workout. You just need to get some rest and let your body recover, but that's easier said than done with a little one who needs round-the-clock attention.

Try to watch your posture, so that you don't end up with backache. I suffered with this quite badly with all of mine as I was permanently carrying and rocking – this takes its toll on your back, particularly when your core is still weak. If you're far enough into your recovery, have been given the all-clear by your doctor and are experiencing back pain, try using a baby carrier or sling to spread the weight and free your arms.

When I first had Harry, I quickly discovered that I had no strength in my legs. When you have a baby you suddenly have to do a lot of standing up from a sitting or squatting position without using your hands because you're holding a child, so your thigh muscles can take a battering. The first time I really noticed it was at bathtime – after I'd dressed Harry for bed on the bathroom floor and picked him up, I suddenly wondered how I'd ever manage to stand up! As with all these things, prevention is better than cure, so try to do a few strengthening exercises along the way to prepare your body. I did maternity yoga whilst pregnant with Belle and Chester, which I found to be a great but very gentle way of strengthening my body.

Episiotomy and stitches ...

Recovering from a difficult birth can be very traumatic for a new mother who already has so much to think about. Even if you didn't end up with any stitches, you will undoubtedly be sore and swollen down below. But if you ended up with an episiotomy (a cut to the vagina to make more room for the baby to come through) or stitches (after tearing or a cut), you will undoubtedly feel very sore. Paracetamol is safe to take whilst you're breastfeeding, so dose yourself up on that for the pain and bathe the area regularly with plain water to keep it clean. You can get specialist ring cushions to sit on so there's no direct pressure on the painful area.

Your stitches will dissolve within a couple of weeks, but to begin with they will feel sore and itchy, particularly when you need to wee and the urine touches the area. You can pour water over the area when you urinate to ease the stinging sensation or use cooled pads to help take away the itch. Leave off your underwear to stop any chafing and allow the area to heal. And don't, whatever you do, drink anything acidic. If anyone offers you a glass of orange juice after you've had your baby, politely decline. You'll thank me for it later!

Postnatal bleeding ...

Having not had a period for nearly a year, you might have forgotten what it's like, but boy does Mother Nature know how to give you a reminder! As soon as you've given birth, you'll start bleeding (it's called lochia) – this will be really heavy to begin with and you might feel gushes when you breastfeed, as your womb contracts with your baby's sucking rhythm. Make sure you have plenty of maternity pads to hand, which are similar to heavy-flow sanitary towels but more absorbent – these are essential for the first few weeks.

The bleeding can continue for up to six weeks, turning from a heavy, bright-red flow to a lighter-brown flow. Don't use tampons until after your six-week check (your regular periods may start any time after that) – use sanitary towels and check them for any blood clots. It's quite normal to pass clots, but it's the size you need to monitor. Anything larger than a 50p should be kept to show the midwife. Equally if the blood flow doesn't show any signs of easing after a few weeks, or you notice a sudden change and that the bleeding suddenly becomes much heavier, then contact your GP. A rush of blood accompanied by dizziness and a fever can be symptomatic of an internal infection.

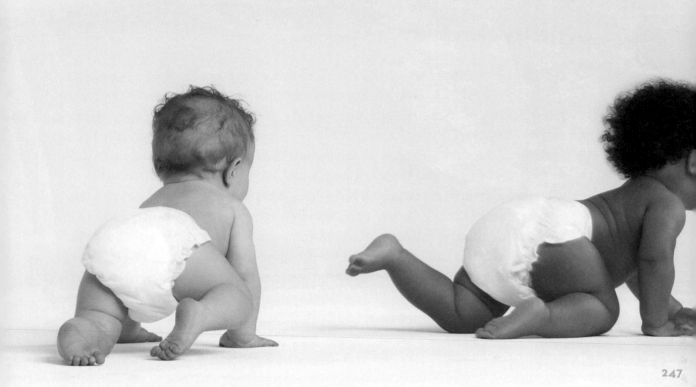

This happened to me after having Harry. I took him for a walk a couple of weeks after bringing him home, suddenly felt a huge gush and knew immediately that the maternity pad didn't stand a chance. I managed to make it to the nearest public toilets, where I passed out. Luckily Dan was with me and phoned an ambulance as I was haemorrhaging quite heavily and later discovered that I did indeed have an infection, which was very treatable with antibiotics. It was a scary moment for everyone involved, but it looked worse than it actually was.

Post-Caesarean care ...

I didn't have a Caesarean section with any of my babies, so I've spoken to my sister and other mummy friends that have and here's their take on how you feel afterwards. Not only do you have all the crazy postpartum hormonal issues to deal with, but you've effectively had major surgery and need to make sure you try to get the recuperation time and support necessary not to end up back in hospital with an infection.

After filming *Celebrity Juice* one night, I got a really scary phone call from my panicked brother-in-law asking me to go straight to Kingston A&E to meet my sister, who'd been carted off in an ambulance with a suspected Caesarean wound infection. Apparently she'd been experiencing rigors, which are intermittent attacks of uncontrollable shaking – a surefire symptom of infection after major surgery. My brother-in-law had been advised to stay at home with three-day-old Lola rather than exposing her to any infections, so he was quite literally left holding the baby! It was the most awful experience and it took all night to run tests and diagnose, but thanks to the brilliant hospital staff, and a strong dose of antibiotics, my sister was on the mend and home within 48 hours. So when I tell you to take this surgery and your recovery very seriously, I speak from first-hand experience about what can go wrong.

After the op Once you come out of theatre with your new baby you'll have to wait for the effects of the epidural or spinal anaesthetic to wear off. It usually takes three to four hours for the feeling to come back in your legs. If you feel woozy, sick or itchy after the operation, there are medicines you can take, so just be sure to talk to the hospital staff about anything abnormal you're experiencing. You'll be given pain relief, which you'll continue to take when you're at home.

You can start breastfeeding straight away – in fact, the sooner you do this, the better. If you had a planned Caesarean, the chances are that everything that happens to a new mother, in particular the milk coming in, might take a bit longer, so if you want to feed your baby, the quicker you kickstart your milk production, the better. You'll also be taught ways to hold your baby to feed to ensure that she isn't pressing down on your wound – the most common is the rugby ball hold (see page 25). Once you get the feeling back in your legs, you'll be encouraged by the nurses to get out of bed – something that you'll be convinced is impossible! – and asked to move around. This is to prevent blood clots and prepare for the catheter being removed. It's important for the catheter to be taken out quickly as apparently your bladder has the memory of a goldfish and can forget how to work if it's left in for too long and has to be retrained. Don't ask me how they do that! Things like coughing or laughing will hurt, and you might feel like you're about to burst your stitches. As for your first bowel movement – childbirth will pale into insignificance compared with how you feel about having to go for your first poo (see page 253) after having a baby! Just drink plenty of water so you don't get constipated and you'll be fine.

I can remember being surprised when I went to visit my sister, how quickly the staff took the dressing off her Caesarean wound. She had the operation at 11am on the Friday morning, and by the Saturday morning the midwife came in and removed the big, sticky, sanitary-type pad that had been covering it, leaving it to heal in the open. Whilst you're in hospital, the nurses will do regular checks on your wound to make sure there's no fluid oozing from it or signs of infection. This is something you'll have to keep up until the midwife visits when you're back at home.

Recovery at home Once you're home keep an eye on your scar for any changes and don't dream of lifting anything heavy or throwing your arms above your head. You'll even need help picking your baby up out of the Moses basket or pram to begin with, as it's best not to bend and lift until a few weeks into your recovery. You can get your wound wet in the shower, but just be gentle when drying it – dab it rather than wipe it. You'll notice the area around your scar feeling numb, which is something I'm told might stay that way for years. You can't drive until you have the OK from your GP, which is usually after six weeks.

It's not all bad, though. As long as you look after yourself for the first few weeks, you'll feel so much stronger by about week three, which isn't bad going after such major surgery. Your scar will most definitely be visible but that will fade slightly with time. As with any scar, once the skin has healed you can try rubbing Vitamin E oil in to reduce the appearance of it.

YOUR BODY AFTER BIRTH

Physical changes ...

During pregnancy and birth, your body will have stretched and changed in more ways than you thought possible – to say nothing of the cellulite, water retention, stretchmarks and jelly-belly! But a lot of these things start to revert to normal in the weeks after you deliver your baby. The first thing you may notice is that your feet look skeletal! You may not have realised how swollen your trotters had become in the third trimester and may have got used to your hands looking like sausages, but there will be a moment when you look down and a) realise you can actually see your feet for the first time in goodness knows how long, and b) they're positively emaciated! They're not, of course – it's just that all the excess water has left your body, leaving you puff-free rather than puf-fy!

> Think of your bodily changes as mummy marks – if they weren't there, your little bundle of joy wouldn't be either.

You're still going to look pregnant after the birth as it takes a while for things to revert to normal. If you're breastfeeding successfully, you'll notice a huge difference quite quickly as you burn calories doing it. It also signals to your uterus to contract back to its original size, pulling your tummy in with it. Don't get me wrong, breastfeeding is not a miracle cure, but it definitely helps. It takes about six weeks for your womb to return to its pre-pregnancy state, so when you go for your six-week check with your GP your progress will be assessed and you'll be advised about what your body can handle in terms of exercise.

I think the main thing to accept is that there's every chance some parts of you will remain forever different after having a baby. Whether it's a scar, a stretch mark, a wider ribcage or bigger feet, don't allow the changes to frustrate or embarrass you, embrace them – your body-image issues mustn't get in the way of happiness.

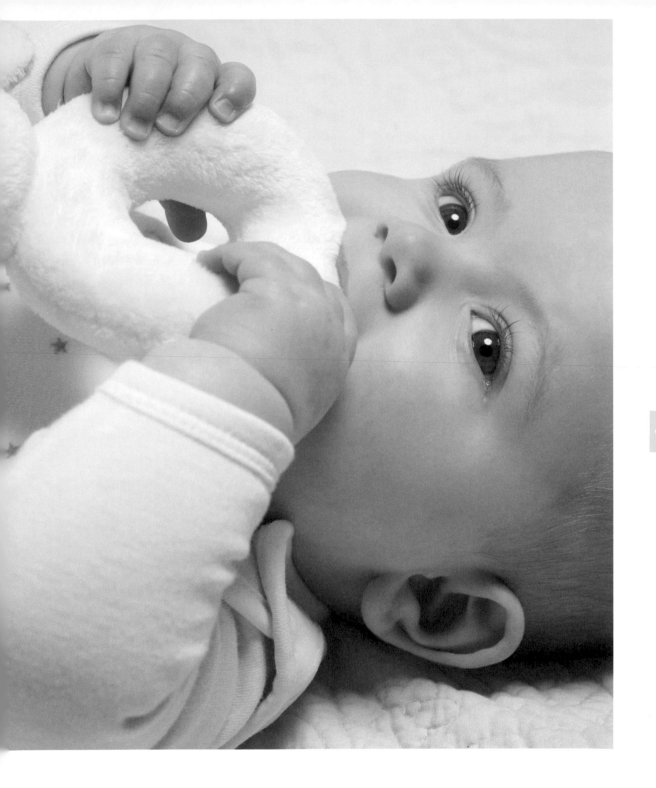

Anaemia ...

It goes without saying that all new mothers feel exhausted and lacking in energy after giving birth, but it's worth getting your iron levels checked to see whether or not you're anaemic, a condition that can leave you feeling even more tired. Anaemia is common because of the blood loss during and after the delivery, but it's easily rectified with iron supplements. Supplements come in liquid or tablet form, but don't take more than the recommended dose or you'll end up constipated, which is the absolute last thing you want!

Vitamin C can also help you to absorb more of the iron in your diet, so that's worth boosting with supplements too. If you had a Caesarean, you'll be particularly susceptible to anaemia.

Bleeding gums and wobbly teeth ...

You're given two free years' dentistry on the NHS when you fall pregnant because your baby will take so much from your calcium reserves that you might suddenly start having dental issues. If you experience anything out of the ordinary, such as your gums bleeding abnormally or your teeth feeling wobbly, make a dental appointment. Falling pregnant and having a baby can literally affect every part of your body! Ensure you're supplementing your Vitamin D and calcium levels enough to prevent this from happening.

Hair loss ...

Because of the abnormally high levels of oestrogen in your body when you are pregnant you don't tend to lose as much hair as usual, making it feel thicker and more luscious. This is fabulous until you give birth, then, at the point when you're feeling your most dowdy, the oestrogen levels dip and you start shedding hair again. In fact you only shed the extra hair you would have shed anyway if you hadn't been pregnant – it just feels like you're going bald as it happens all at once after you give birth. Nature can be cruel!

Toilet trouble ...

Going for a pee The thought of going to the toilet after giving birth can be almost as traumatic as the thought of having another baby! It can really sting. If it's really bad, pour water over the area as you pee, or copy one of my mummy friends, who used to run a little bath and go in it to ease the pain. Needs must!

Your first poo So now onto your first proper bowel movement! There will come a moment where you'll sit and contemplate how it's even going to be possible, given your stitches and piles, but it is! If I can tell you anything comforting it's that you will achieve it and it won't be anywhere near as bad as you thought. Don't put it off or the stools will harden, making it even more difficult. You need to avoid constipation at all costs, so make sure you're eating proper, fibre-packed meals, and if you're on medication where constipation is a side effect, drink some prune juice!

Now I'm going to pass on a tip that a very kind midwife told me. It's not glamorous but it may help. When you're on the loo, lean forward with your elbows on your knees – picture a man reading a newspaper on a toilet. Apparently this puts your body in the optimum position to do your business!

Bladder incontinence Because of all the pressure on your bladder during pregnancy and birth, it's likely you'll experience a leaky bladder if you cough, sneeze or laugh. The only way you can combat this is by doing pelvic floor exercises (see page 265) and if these don't work, you might need to see a physiotherapist. Unless you have a pelvic floor of steel, you'll always be aware of it. Like when your toddler begs you to go on the trampoline and after a couple of bounces you're reminded you're not as firm as you once were!

Piles If you suffered from piles during pregnancy, the strain and pressure of giving birth might have made these worse. They will go down, but make sure you're getting all the fibre you need to avoid getting constipated. If you had stitches, the rubber ring you bought to sit on will help, too (see page 246). I know, it's a nightmare! But just look at that beautiful baby ... again!

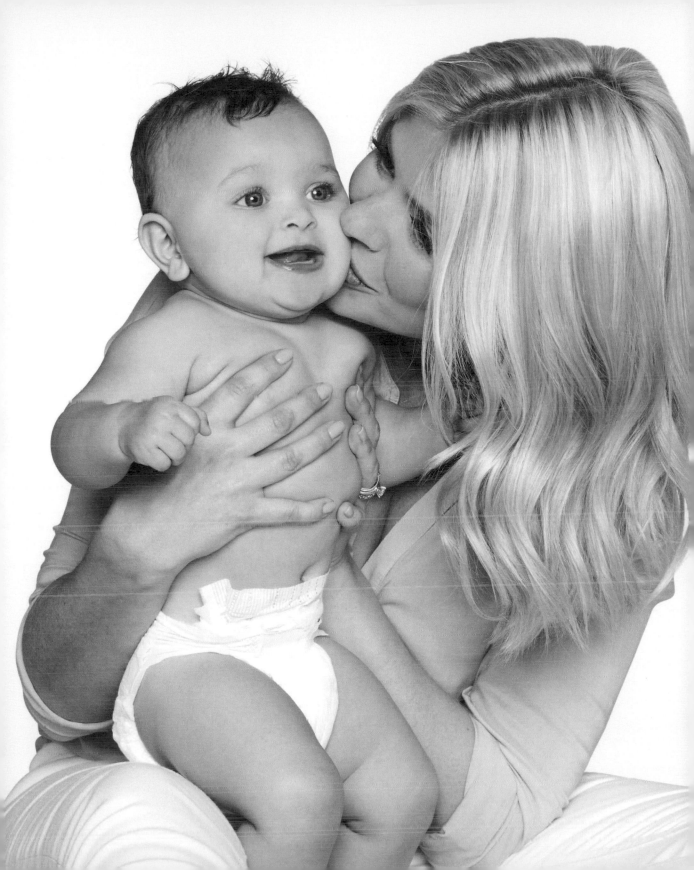

Breastfeeding issues ...

You'll find lots of info on breastfeeding trouble in the Feeding chapter (see pages 67–9), but these are a few other things you might experience when you're breastfeeding that don't directly impact on getting milk into your baby – they're just a bit rubbish for you!

Uterine cramps It's usual for you to feel period-pain-type cramps as you breastfeed, because the rhythmic sucking motion causes your womb to contract. This is a good thing as it's a sign that your body's trying to get back to normal. You might also notice you bleed more as you feed, which again is a good sign that everything is on the move.

Engorgement Whilst you're waiting for your milk to come in, you can feel very poorly with a high fever, the shivers and then swollen, painful breasts. You can take paracetamol whilst you're breastfeeding for the pain, so do that and then use hot flannels or have a warm bath to reduce the inflammation and, if you can bear it, put your baby on the breast as that's the best way to release some pressure and clear any blocked ducts. I had a lot of milk come in with Belle, but because she was premature and so tiny she couldn't empty them fully at each feed, which left me feeling quite uncomfortable sometimes. If I was in pain after a feed, I found lying in a warm bath released the pressure, as some of the unused milk would make its way into the bath.

Sore nipples Slather on the lanolin cream, before and after feeding. Your baby can feed through it, so keep your nipples coated at all times. You can also try nipple shields if they're really sore (see page 67).

Leaky boobs For the first month or so, whilst your milk production is adapting to how much your baby needs, you might experience very leaky boobs. Breast pads, breast pads, breast pads! I can remember going through this phase with all of mine, where if I didn't get a pad on quick enough I'd end up with a wet shirt in seconds, particularly early on when the milk doesn't just drip out, but spurts. Nightmare! This irregular, erratic leaking only happens until your milk production settles down, and then you can stop buying pads in bulk!

Newfound hunger Breastfeeding makes you hungry – fact! It's because of all the energy you're burning up producing milk, which is why you lose some of your baby weight in the early feeding days. Make sure you have plenty of healthy foods in the house to snack on so you don't plough your way through the biscuit tin, and drink plenty of water. I drank gallons of water whilst I was breastfeeding, because I found as soon as I started it felt like I hadn't had a drink for days!

Empty boobs When you make the decision to stop breastfeeding and you stop producing milk, I'm going to be very honest with you and say that your breasts will look different to how you remember them. Now hear this, and hear me well … your breasts were put there to feed your child. You have done this and given her the best start in life. This is a miracle and something that you should be incredibly proud of.

I've breastfed all three of my children and in 2016 was asked to be the cover girl on the last ever edition of *FHM* magazine with full cleavage on show. Despite feeling nervous, off I went to the photoshoot with my extremely non-youthful, but all-mine, boobs. One of the main reasons I did it was because I wanted to fly the flag for postnatal women and their bodies. Now go forth and burn your bra! Actually on second thoughts, keep a tight hold on that bra, because that's your best friend for life!

On the plus side, once you stop producing milk your body lets go of the little fat reserves it's been holding onto whilst you were feeding, so you might find you suddenly drop a bit more baby weight – every cloud – even if it is from your boobs!

Feeding struggle and guilt Breastfeeding is an art! Don't despair. It's definitely worth persevering with but equally you know when it's time to stop, whether that's after a successful stint of breastfeeding or as a result of it having been a continuous struggle. Don't let anyone make you feel guilty – and you *will* come across these people, whether they are healthcare professionals or friends and family. Remember, this is your baby, your life and your decision. End of story! And, ultimately, could you walk into the office and pick out those who were breastfed as babies and those who definitely weren't? Of course you couldn't! But could you tell which people had a loving and happy childhood and grew into well-rounded adults? Of course you could. And that's where your priorities should lie.

Breastfeeding after alcohol …

One unit of alcohol (a small glass of wine or half a pint of lager) will take two hours to leave the bloodstream. The choice is yours. If you do decide to have a glass of wine, this doesn't make you a bad mum; just make sure you have it soon after a completed feed so that it's got enough time to get out of your system before the next feed. Everything I've read and been told suggests that babies don't take as much milk if there's alcohol in it so you risk disrupting their feeds, which then has a knock-on effect for them becoming fussy and not sleeping as well. Alcohol also has a negative effect on your letdown reflex, so you risk messing with the milk you have fought so hard to establish.

My advice is if your baby is happy to take milk from a bottle, have a glass of wine or two, and pump and dump (that is, express your milk, then throw it away), even though you'll cry as the liquid gold pours down the sink! A night off might just be the thing you need. However, go gently! Being hungover with small children is no fun whatsoever, and you will ask yourself the next day whether it was really worth it! But the odd glass of wine once in a while as a treat is something you absolutely shouldn't be afraid of!

YOUR MENTAL STATE AFTER HAVING A BABY

Falling in love with your baby ...

You will feel such euphoria at having given birth successfully. No matter how hard or traumatic the experience, the fact that you both came out the other side, healthy and complete, will hopefully give you such a feeling of achievement. All my labours were very different, but that moment when you look into your child's eyes for the first time and that feeling of love wooshes into every part of your being was the same for all of them. However, if like some women you don't feel this rush of love immediately, don't give yourself a tough time. Be open with your partner about it, otherwise it will feel like some horrible secret or that in some way you're a bad person for not feeling instant love for your baby.

The truth is, it happens to us all at different times because everyone is different. There also might be a chemical reason for you not connecting immediately. Any stress or fear you experienced during labour will have increased the levels of cortisol (the stress hormone) in your body, blocking the rush of oxytocin (the love hormone), so is it any wonder you don't know what to feel?

Hormonal wooooosh of emotion ...

Giving birth is a tiring and stressful process, no matter how good your experience, but when you add in all the emotions around meeting your baby for the first time, the stress of doing a job you've never done before and the responsibility of being that baby's lifeline, on top of all the crazy hormones rushing around your body, is it any wonder you're tearful?! Go easy on yourself. There's been so much change and everything's happening at once. It would be strange if you didn't feel weepy.

The best piece of advice I can share is to give in to all that emotion and don't hide it away. I used to announce quite frequently that 'I'm going to have a cry now' and promptly burst into tears. It's a scientific fact that the physical release of tears relieves stress. You're allowed to have a little cry. It's not always a sign you're not coping – in fact, it's as much a sign that you

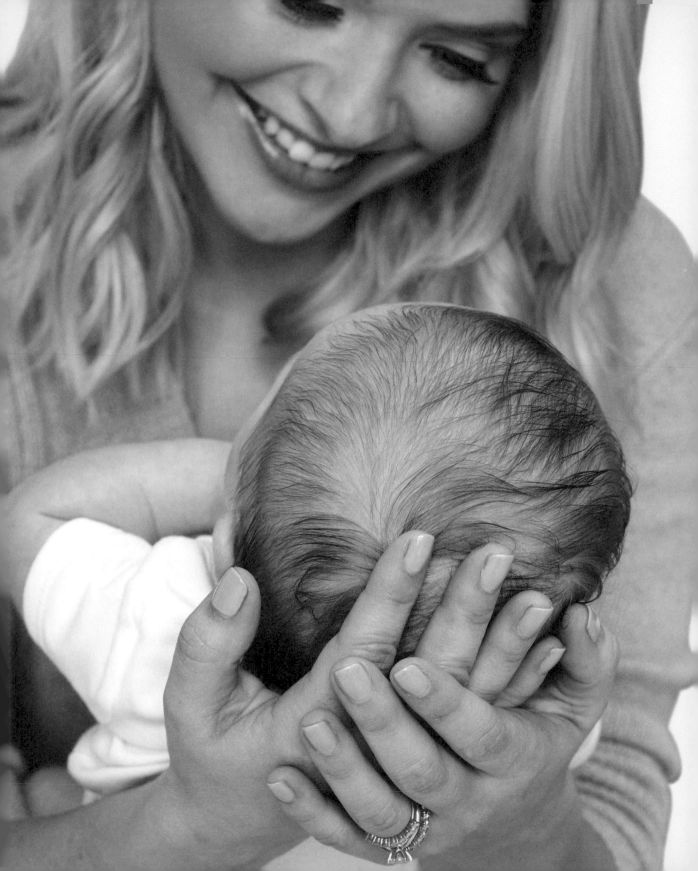

are coping and accepting all the changes to your life and your body. As with everything, if you're feeling tearful and overwhelmed, it's just a phase and it won't last forever. I was particularly emotional with Chester, partly because we had such a tough start due to his reflux and feeding issues. I think it was magnified because he was my third child, so I'd been so confident I knew the ropes that when my little curve ball arrived I became frustrated and despairing, bursting into tears as soon as anyone gave me a cuddle. Know that it's all going to be all right. Right now you're exhausted and not thinking straight, but think what you'd tell yourself if you popped in to visit you and your baby for the first time. Take each day as it comes and ask for help. It takes time, but you'll feel back to your old self in no time. I guarantee it!

The baby blues …

You might experience the baby blues in the first week after giving birth, due to the hormonal changes taking place in your body. These can affect your state of mind, making you feel tearful and irritable, or leave you feeling concerned about your baby all the time. This is completely natural. Just make sure you tell your family how you are feeling. I always find I feel much better once I've shared my thoughts and worries. Sometimes just saying the words out loud can make you feel better. The baby blues will soon pass once your hormones level out and you get used to this brand new little person being in your life.

Postnatal depression and postnatal psychosis …

Postnatal depression is different, in that it's unlikely to get better without help. Whereas the baby blues occur during the first week after birth, postnatal depression can be an ongoing illness that gets worse without intervention. As the days and weeks go by, most mummies can feel fed up, like they're on an ever-turning not-so-merry-go-round of feeding, nappy changing and feeding. This is normal. Along with all the positives, coping with a new baby can be frustrating, overwhelming, exhausting and terribly emotional. But if you feel it is more than this and you really can't cope, reach out to somebody – your partner, a midwife, a friend, a relative or a GP, as you might have postnatal depression.

Be comforted by the fact that postnatal depression is a common condition and not your fault. It's a chemical reaction in your brain to all the changes, but it can be treated. There is a much rarer but more serious level of postnatal depression, called postnatal psychosis. Sadly, more often than not, if you have it, you won't know that anything's wrong. Ensure your family know about this condition and can recognise the signs, so that they can get the correct psychiatric help for you as it can be dangerous for you and your baby. If you need help with any of these conditions, there are lots of very helpful websites (see page 280), but I'd definitely speak to a medical professional first.

A new baby in the house can be an enormous pressure on everyone.

New dads can also suffer from postnatal depression. Keep an eye on each other for developing symptoms such as irritability, anxiety, changes in appetite and general down behaviour. Dads can feel emotionally and financially stressed, and it doesn't help that all mum's time has suddenly been taken up by the baby, and over time a dad can feel pushed out as he's unable to participate in the relationship much in the early days. This is where giving your partner a daily responsibility like doing one of the night feeds or bathtime is great. Not only does it help you, but the responsibility will boost his confidence as a new father and help him to bond with the baby.

Exhaustion …

The end of your pregnancy was exhausting, as were labour and delivery, and now you have this little bundle of joy who wants to feed all night! Often the excitement surrounding your new arrival will give you strength and energy, but once the first few weeks are over, and perhaps your partner has gone back to work, the novelty might wear off, leaving you with the reality of no sleep and a mountain of washing. The only advice I can give here is to ask for help, even if it's just getting a friend over after a feed so you can get your head down for an hour, or asking your partner to look after the baby once he gets home from work so you can go to bed. Do what you have to in order to get by. Who cares if nothing's ironed or there are dirty dishes? As long as your environment is hygienic, what does a bit of mess matter?! Do an online order, or ask someone to go shopping for oven- or microwave-ready meals. Sleep when your baby sleeps. Remember, this is just a phase which will pass quicker than you think!

If you're anything like me and most new mums on the planet, you'll get to a point where your baby cries out in the night for the third or fourth time and you stir, thinking, 'I just can't get up.' You're so exhausted, you can't even swing your legs out of bed. Well, here's something that worked for me, and I still do it to this day when my alarm goes off at unsociable o'clock! I learnt it when I was practising yoga. At the end of the session, when you're completely zonked out and lying on the floor wondering how you're ever going to get up, the yoga teacher would say wiggle your toes, then your fingers, take two deep breaths in, then on the third breath, think, 'Right, I'm going to get up on this breath,' and I'd suddenly feel a surge of energy to get up. Try it!

Confidence boost ...

Knowing that are you loved unconditionally and needed by your baby can make you feel ten feet tall – and where you might have lacked confidence before, you suddenly become brave. Use this surge in confidence to your advantage: approach another mum in the park for a chat or be more driven when you return to work. Before children your life might have been unbalanced and perhaps you lost sight of what was important. Becoming a mother can help you to prioritise differently. Since being a mum, I'm better at my job because a) it's made me more time-efficient, and b) I only focus on things that really matter.

And everything else ...

Be prepared for your attitude to change! You might become relaxed about things you used to sweat about, like punctuality. On the flip side you might become militant about routine and making sure the washing is done before it's erupting over the top of the basket. You'll probably become more patient with people who have children. You'll stop living for the next social event and start living for the moment, as every second spent with your child is precious.

You might become super-protective of your entire family, including your parents, because it's only after having your own child that you know how it feels to be willing to give your life for someone. Things like flying, which had never bothered me before, now scared the living daylights out of me when taking my children. This was well and truly tested with Harry when he came to the *X Factor*'s judges' houses with me at two months old – with every air mile we collected I grew another grey hair! Being convinced I was going to leave them orphaned was one of the irrational thoughts I experienced, so don't be surprised if you start to have very odd thoughts, too!

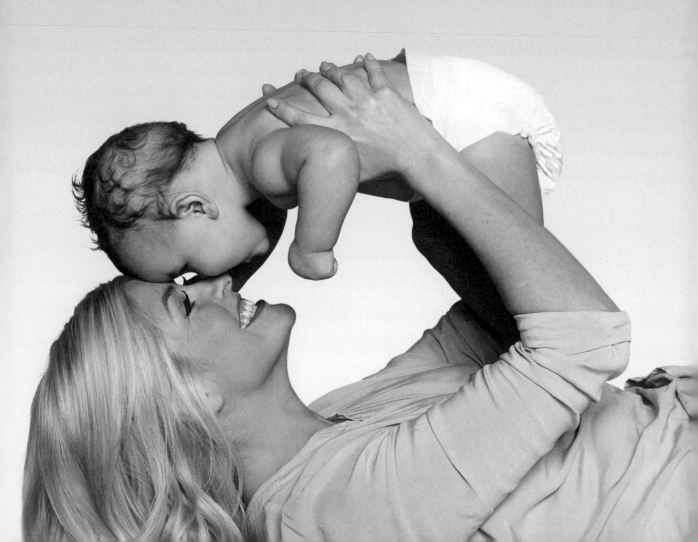

02 Life after having a baby

There's no going back now, and why would you want to?! Your baby is in your arms and you're embarking on life as a new family, which can be both weird and wonderful all at once!

Once you're out of the initial newborn frenzy, you might be wondering how to squeeze some more exercise into your routine so you can start to feel a bit more like you again. My advice here would be to take it slow! A little goes a long way, and tiring yourself out through the gym or unrealistic dieting will put a strain on everything. Eat healthily, take walks with the pram and spend any spare moments on yourself or making the most of your new little family.

POST-BIRTH TO-DO LIST

Pelvic floor and abdominal exercises Your pelvic floor muscles support your bladder and your bowel, and with all the pressure put on them during pregnancy and labour they can become weak and, at worst, leave you incontinent. I can remember the midwife ending every pregnancy appointment with a reminder to keep my pelvic floor strong or I'd regret it, and she was right!

If you're the other side of giving birth and experiencing embarrassing leaks, it's not too late to start and you will notice a difference within a couple of months. You know which muscles I'm talking about if you squeeze and stop your urine flow halfway through. Remember that movement and repeat it, increasing the length of time you hold the squeeze as the days and weeks go by. You don't have to be on the loo to do it. Once you get used to the sensation, you can do it anywhere, any time! I always found that doing it whilst cleaning my teeth morning and night was the easiest way to remember.

Your ever-growing baby can cause your abdominal muscles to move apart and weaken. After you've given birth, you can feel the gap in between your ribs for a few months, and there are exercises you can do to encourage the muscles to move back together once you've had the all-clear from your GP.

Exercising to lose your jelly-belly Be careful about doing too much until you've had the all-clear from your GP at your six-week check. Chances are you will have been too busy with a certain little person to spend hours down at the gym anyway, but it's important that you don't overdo it before your body has recovered properly from the delivery. Begin with getting out with your baby for short walks. It's very easy to feel cooped up in the house after you first come home, so getting some fresh air and a little bit of exercise will do wonders for clearing the cobwebs away.

Foods to eat to lose the baby weight If you're breastfeeding successfully, you're burning calories by doing it. You'll be hungry, though, so just make sure you're getting healthy foods and that all the main food groups are represented: proteins, vegetables, fruits, grains and low-fat dairy products – you don't want to be going on any crazy diets where you're cutting out carbs when you need all your strength to take care of your baby.

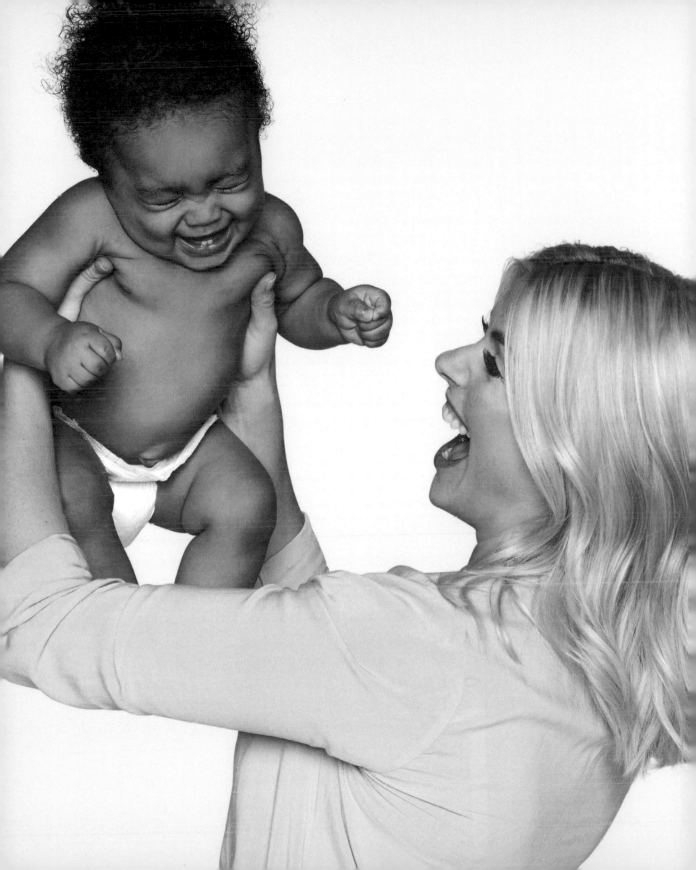

YOUR OTHER HALF

The bond with your partner …

Dan and I are lucky in that our children have brought us closer together than ever. I thought getting married was the be-all and end-all when it came to feeling like a forever team, but having Harry, then Belle and now Chester has cemented us beyond belief. I think for men, sometimes just watching you go through labour and feeling so relieved they never have to go through that can lead to a newfound respect and admiration for your strength and resilience.

Don't get me wrong, there have been times when we've both been absolutely exhausted by work pressures and children, taking it in turns to be up through the night, and we've been irritable with each other, but we're all human. Give yourself and each other a break and allow one another to make mistakes. Don't jump on those small things that irritate you about each other just because you're tired. Just acknowledge that these early days and months and years are going to test you, but ultimately it's a test that will make you stronger as a couple.

As long as you keep talking and try to make time for the two of you – if only a two-minute chat at bedtime – your relationship will be fine. You might see a whole new side to your partner that you've never witnessed before either, and he will feel the same about you. When you're holding the baby and pacing the room, utterly exhausted, and your partner comes home from work and takes over, just seeing the qualities in him of being a good, nurturing father and him seeing you as a good mother can be really attractive. Doing things together with the baby means that you're spending time together, and the fact that you're both exhausted, but sharing the experience, will keep you close without too much effort. Then once you feel confident enough to leave your baby with someone you trust, pop down the road for a quick bite to eat. You'll be surprised how weird it feels, being just the two of you again – you'll probably spend the whole time talking about your gorgeous baby anyway!

Resuming your sex life ...

In your own time The official advice is to wait for at least six weeks after giving birth before you start having sex again. But essentially, you know when you are ready. Just make sure it's your decision and what you really want. If you've had a difficult delivery (episiotomy, stitches or a Caesarean), you'll probably want to wait longer to give your body the recovery time it needs. If you have sex too early, you can put your wounds at risk of infection. Whatever you decide, just make sure you talk to your partner about how you are feeling.

Your reason for not wanting to have sex might not be anything more than exhaustion, which is perfectly valid. You also might be feeling insecure about your body: 'Will my partner still be turned on by my new wobbles and some-what altered lady bits?!' Having been faced with this situation three times, I can honestly hand on heart say that men do not think in the same way as us, at all. And, if anything, at this moment, they love you more than ever. It's also worth knowing that Mother Nature does something really cruel at this time. To make sure we form a strong bond with our babies, it's been medically proven that all our love hormones are directed towards that baby, leaving our partners out of the equation. It's also been scientifically proven that it remains this way for the first 18 months of your baby's life. So don't, for goodness sake, start making life-changing decisions about how you must not love your partner any more because you can't face having sex with him, as actually it could just be down to that wonderful, but not always helpful, Mother Nature!

Communicate When it comes to your partner and your sex life, just keep talking about it. Talk about doing it. Talk about not doing it. Talk about how you're too tired to do it. Talk about how everyone else is doing it. And at that point talk about the fact that everyone else is talking about doing it rather than actually doing it! Communication is key to your partner understanding and empathising with everything you're going through, but in particular about how your relationship has changed and how you feel about him. He's not the one who went through a pregnancy and delivery, so he may be ready and willing to have sex whenever you give the green light, but however long that takes, talking to each other as you go along will alleviate any build-up of frustration.

I must say, though, that there is no doubt in my mind that if you really want to feel like you again, it's not about losing weight. It's not about having your first massive blow-out night on the white wine, it is about feeling loved and sexy and having a night with your man.

Vaginal issues You'll probably find you need extra lubrication following childbirth, especially if you're breastfeeding, due to the drop in oestrogen levels after giving birth. You might also find that your vagina is more sensitive or that it's been stretched during delivery, or tightened when stitched. Things might have moved around inside too, feeling lower or higher than they were. Ultimately, though, sex shouldn't be painful after having a baby, so if you're experiencing pain, make an appointment with your GP – and if you're not wanting to fall pregnant again any time soon, make sure you're on the right contraception for you (see below).

Watch out – you're fertile There is a school of thought that says you're less fertile whilst you're exclusively breastfeeding – it's impossible to know exactly how long that will last but it's definitely not something I would have felt comfortable relying on as a contraceptive! If you don't want to fall pregnant again right away (which I imagine will be the last thing on your mind), you should know that you can get pregnant as soon as two to three weeks after giving birth. Don't be thinking that you're safe until your periods start up again, because you will have ovulated before your period begins, so could already be pregnant if you haven't taken precautions. Speak to your GP about the best form of contraception for you.

BIG BROTHERS AND SISTERS

If you're a mummy already, you might find life with your second baby quite different to the first time round. As mummy to both, you'll be torn between wanting to give the new baby all the time and love you gave your first-born, and trying to prevent your other child(ren) from feeling left out or replaced.

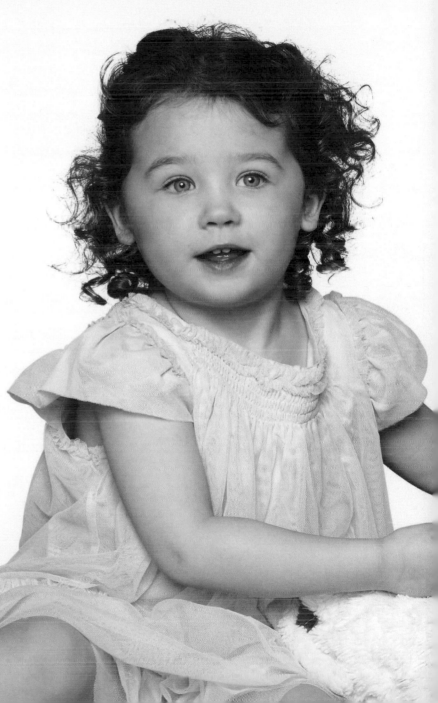

When I had Belle I made sure I had a little gift for Harry in my hospital bag, so that when he came to visit us for the first time, in his eyes, the baby had bought him a present. I did exactly the same when Chester was born, with Harry and Belle. Another thing you can do is to ask grandparents and friends to focus their attention on the other children when they are in the room, rather than gushing over the baby.

I think your partner's help is key when you bring a second baby home. He will need to do more of the feeds and help with the other children, particularly in the early days. Once your new baby starts to give more back, in terms of smiles, etc., siblings should start to relax. It's the first couple of months, where the new baby needs every second of your attention to survive, that are tough for the others, so try to include them as much as possible. Harry was six when Chester was born, so he was far more receptive to helping, bringing me clean nappies, etc., which made him feel part of Chester's life.

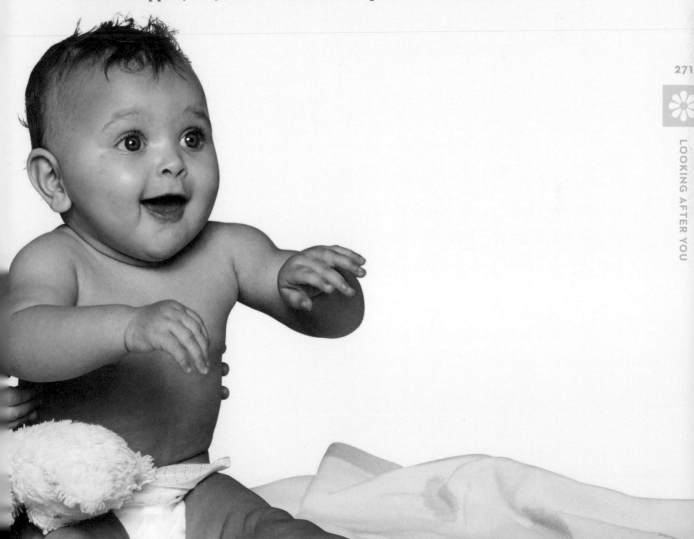

03 Support for you and your new baby

Support comes in two forms, emotional and physical, and I would say accept both in swathes! You can never have too much help when you have a baby, whether it be asking your in-laws to take over from your own mum when she's decided to go home, pumping your mummy friends for advice or just having a good whinge. There's no substitute for feeling loved and supported, and actually being reminded there's probably another mummy a couple of doors down from you going through the exact same thing can be the most comforting thing of all.

If you don't have enough support around you at this time, find out what services are in your local area. In fact, sometimes it's easier to accept help and advice from a stranger if you feel weighed down or overwhelmed by the advice coming from family and friends.

FAMILY AND FRIENDS

Help at home ...

If your partner is off work, great; if not, try to find someone who can be on hand to stay and help, or visit often, for the first couple of weeks. Whoever it is, ask them to fill up the freezer. If someone offers to bring you a fish pie instead of flowers, bite their hand off! And whether you or your partner have OCD tendencies or not, ignore the state of the house. Your new baby is your new priority, so as long as she's clean and fed, the rest can wait.

Grandparents ...

Grandparents can be a complete godsend in terms of extra love and support once you're home. I've watched with my own family how the bond has grown between all of my children and their grandparents, and it melts your heart to see how much the kids love them. I guess the biggest thing to remember with grandparents, particularly if, like me, you have ones who are willing and able to help out, is not to take advantage of their generosity. It's easier said than done when we all have busy lives, but try not to take too much, or you risk bad feeling.

The other problem you can encounter is an overbearing grandparent, particularly in the early days with your first child where you might feel overwhelmed by their advice and criticism. The best thing to do in this instance is to try to explain how you feel, or get your partner to! More often than not, the grandparent in question is just trying to be helpful and hasn't realised the advice is making you feel inadequate or anxious. Grandparents have every right to want to play a key role in their grandchildren's lives, but it can become a little overwhelming and you are well within your rights to pull back a bit and do what's right for you and your baby.

Here's some advice: when it comes to advice, it's totally natural for people to want to pass it on, and it's totally natural for you to want to seek it, but just be careful that the advice doesn't have an adverse effect on your confidence and what you innately know is best for you and your baby.

Friends and visitors ...

Don't fall into the trap of making sure your baby is fed and sleeping soundly so your visitors get lovely sleepy cuddles, whilst you race round and make tea for everyone, only for them to leave right at the time your baby is screaming for a feed. Far better that they take the baby out and you catch up on sleep or whatever you feel up to – even if it's the last three episodes of *Corrie* you recorded!

One thing I think is crucial in the early days is to keep your baby cocooned in as healthy an environment as possible. Ask visitors to let you know if they're feeling unwell, even if it's just a cold, so you can reschedule. People probably will, but ask everyone to wash their hands before holding the baby – particularly children. Of course, being exposed to germs will help build your baby's immune system, but not this early. New babies are very susceptible to illness, so far better not to expose them if you don't have to.

Connect with other mums ...

Becoming a mum automatically connects you with every other mother on the planet. It doesn't matter who you are, where you've come from or what you have, you have all been through and continue to go through the unifying experience of motherhood, and it can be a wonderful comfort. Don't be shy to connect with other mums when you're out and about. The chances are, the mum sitting on the other end of the bench with the dark circles is as desperate as you to speak to a fellow adult for ten minutes about being up all night and exhausted.

There are so many places to meet other mums. NCT groups can be great if you're one of the lucky ones who kept in touch with one or more of the girls. If you weren't so lucky, try going to other mum and baby groups (see pages 227–31).

Parenting is the same – whatever your family unit Whether you're a parent in a heterosexual relationship, a same-sex relationship or if you're a single parent, your role is the same. So long as your baby is loved and cared for to the best of your ability, you will both be fine. The most important thing is your support network, and making sure you get the help and answers you need, when you need them.

Mummy friendship can be invaluable. I would put my baby down whilst my husband babysat for us, then I'd pop down the road and sit for my friend whilst she and her husband went out. They would return the favour, meaning both sets of parents would get a much-needed break.

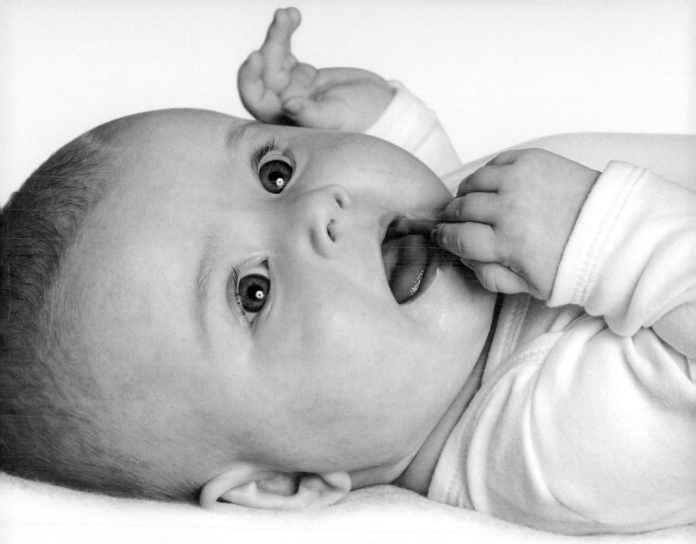

OUTSIDE HELP

Health visitors ...

Your health visitor will take over from the midwives about ten days after the birth. Being a trained nurse or midwife herself, she will have a wealth of baby knowledge, so don't be afraid to make a list of queries and ask her advice. During her visits she'll check you and your baby over for any health problems and will talk you through various appointments you need to make, such as your six-week check and your baby's vaccinations, and where and when your baby should be weighed and measured. Your health visitor will be available to you up until your child reaches five years old.

Support groups ...

There are plenty of dedicated new parent services that offer support and advice. Your local child health clinic, children's centre and Family Information Service together can cover any questions or concerns you might have. There are also dedicated support groups if you're a single parent or if your child has special needs (see page 281). You can find all of these on the NHS website, and your health visitor should also be able to advise.

Doulas ...

The official definition of a doula is a woman who gives support, help and advice to another woman during pregnancy and during and after birth. If you're worried about your support network, and it's financially feasible, finding a doula to help you through it all could be the answer for you.

Maternity nurses – day and/or night ...

If you're in a financial position to do so you can hire maternity nurses, who specialise in looking after newborns. Depending on the level of care you require, they are available to live in around the clock or you may just want someone to do the nights for the first few weeks to get the baby into some good patterns whilst you recover. You work out together what you'd like to achieve by the time she leaves, in terms of a realistic routine, and after she goes you'll have enough confidence to pick up the reins and go it alone. A friend of mine who was having twins asked friends and family not to buy her any baby presents but instead put money towards her being able to hire a night nurse one night a week, so that she knew she would at least be having one decent night's sleep in every seven!

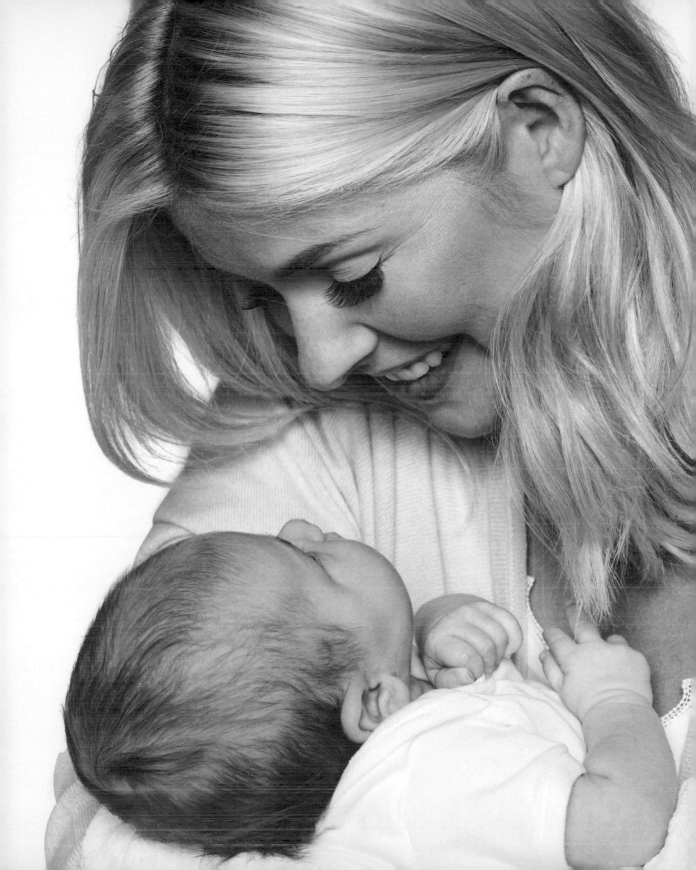

Summary Life as a new mum can be a rollercoaster of emotions and experiences. This mummy job is as new to you as the world is to your baby, and the only thing you can do is take it day by day, learning and growing together as you go. You can do this, and I promise that you will feel like you again very soon!

A new baby in the family can strengthen bonds like nothing else. Enjoy these times, celebrate each other and welcome the future ...

SOME EXTRA ADVICE

Medicines to try …

There are many baby-suitable medicines on the market, and I dare say many more coming through. Here are a few you can look for if you don't know where to start. Always check that any medicines you use are age-appropriate for your baby, and follow the recommended dosage guidelines.

For colic and gripe

- Dentinox
- Gripe water
- Infacol

For pain relief

- Infant ibuprofen (big supermarkets and health stores have their own brands; popular independent brands include Nurofen)
- Infant paracetamol (big supermarkets and health stores have their own brands; popular independent brands include Calpol)

For reflux

- Prescribed medicines from your GP
- Try lactose-free milk, e.g. Nurtamigen Lipil Formula

For teething

- Anbesol
- Homeopathic teething powders
- Teething gels
- Teething granules
- Teething rings

More information …

General

- Doulas – www.doula.org.uk
- Postnatal depression and psychosis – Mind (www.mind.org.uk) and PANDAS (www.pandasfoundation.org.uk)

- Registering your baby – www.gov.uk/register-offices
- Registering your baby with a GP – www.nhs.uk (search services and support for new parents)
- Reusable nappies – www.goreal.org.uk

Breastfeeding organisations

There are a lot of breastfeeding helplines out there, so do some research online. Here are a few:

- Association of Breastfeeding Mothers (abm.me.uk)
- Breastfeeding Network (www.breastfeedingnetwork.org.uk)
- La Leche League (www.laleche.org.uk)

Mum forums and advice websites

- Baby Centre (www.babycentre.co.uk)
- Lullaby Trust (www.lullabytrust.org.uk)
- Mumsnet (www.mumsnet.com)
- Netmums (www.netmums.com)

Support

- Financial support – www.gov.uk/contact-child-benefit-office
- For parents whose children may need social care – Family Rights Group (www.frg.org.uk)
- For parents with disabled children – Contact a Family (www.cafamily.org.uk)
- For single parents – Gingerbread (www.gingerbread.org.uk)

And a few things that worked for me …

- Activity toy – Fisher-Price Jumperoo (expensive but worth it, and has been loved by all three of my babies!)
- Chester's bedside cot – SnuzPod^2 Bedside Crib 3-in-1
- High chair (that comes close to the table) – Tripp Trapp
- Nipple shields – Medela
- Sleeping bags – Grobag and Love to Dream Swaddle (which allows the hands to be above the head)

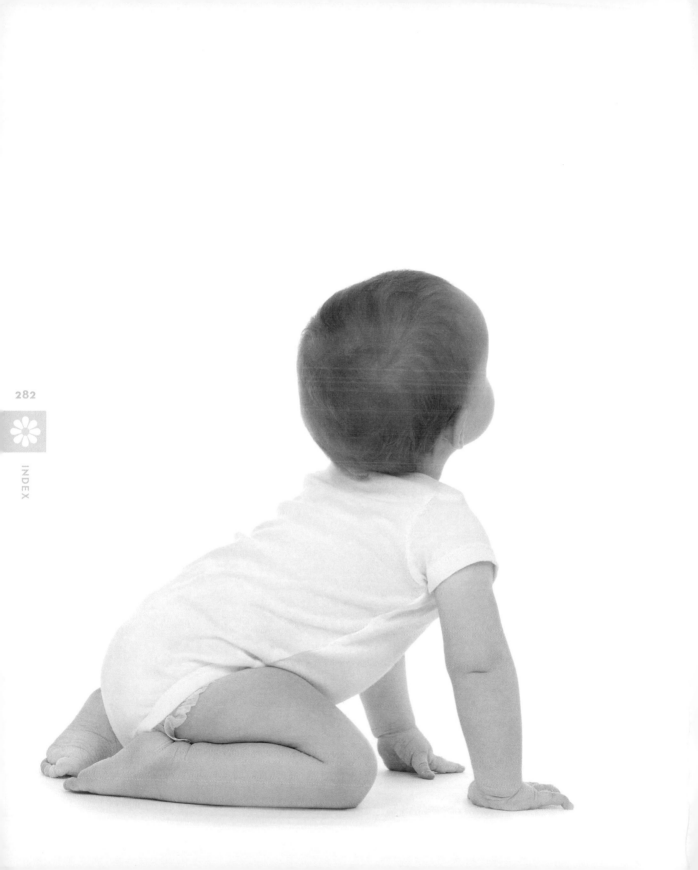

Index

Where to begin with the thank yous for this book?!

First, my thanks go to an incredible mum and wonderful person … my sister Kelly. Without Kelly, not only would this book not have been possible, but during all those motherhood moments where I found myself lost or unsure she'd either have the answer or, if not, she'd just listen and always be there with a cup of tea and a cuddle. We've always been close: playing together as children; going out together as teenagers; buying our first flat together; writing the *School for Stars* children's books together – and now this. She has been a fundamental part of making this pipe-dream a reality, turning all my thoughts into sentences on the page. This book is something we both feel unbelievably proud of together, but as an individual I'm so proud of how Kelly has gone from being my big sis, who used to write and read me her own fairy tales, to becoming the brilliant author she is today.

The next huge thank you goes to my own mother. Mum, you are my inspiration for this book. Your unconditional love has guided and shaped two girls, who now hope to guide so many others. And Dad, thank you too. You are a solid and grounded family man who taught us always to see the light at the end of the tunnel and to keep it shining.

To my husband Dan, thank you for our family. I couldn't have wished for more … you've made my own fairy tale come true.

There are so many other people who helped to get this book off the ground. Thank you to Emily, Claire, Mary, Rowan and everyone at James Grant for all your hard work and unwavering support.

Also thanks to the whole publishing team at HarperCollins – particularly *editor* Emily, *creative* Claire and *listener* Lucy – for believing in our idea and working so hard to make it a reality. Your enthusiasm, patience and determination to read our minds has made this project a pleasure from start to finish.

And now, to all the scrumptious babies who allowed us to feature your beautiful faces in the book: thank you to my two gorgeous nieces – my *smiley cover-girl* Darcy and *adorable toddler* Lola. And to all the other babies: Stacy, Milo, Phoebe, Aitana, Bethan, Ted, Max, Luca, Talah, Evie, James and Emma (and their parents for giving their blessing!). You all behaved impeccably considering it was your first photoshoot. Whoever said never work with children clearly hadn't met you lot! Thanks, too, to the lovely breastfeeding mum Sabrina and baby Alvin, who were both completely unflappable.

And finally . . . thank you to you, my fellow mum, for picking up this book and trusting me to hold your hand through one of the most important times of your life. This is just the beginning, so stay calm and talk things through with friends and loved ones … a lot! Talking helps, but so does listening – and the loudest voice you should listen to is your own. Remember: turn on intuition and switch off fear. Your instinct as a mum will always guide you well and keep you on the track that's right for you and your baby. Good luck with everything!

Big love,

x

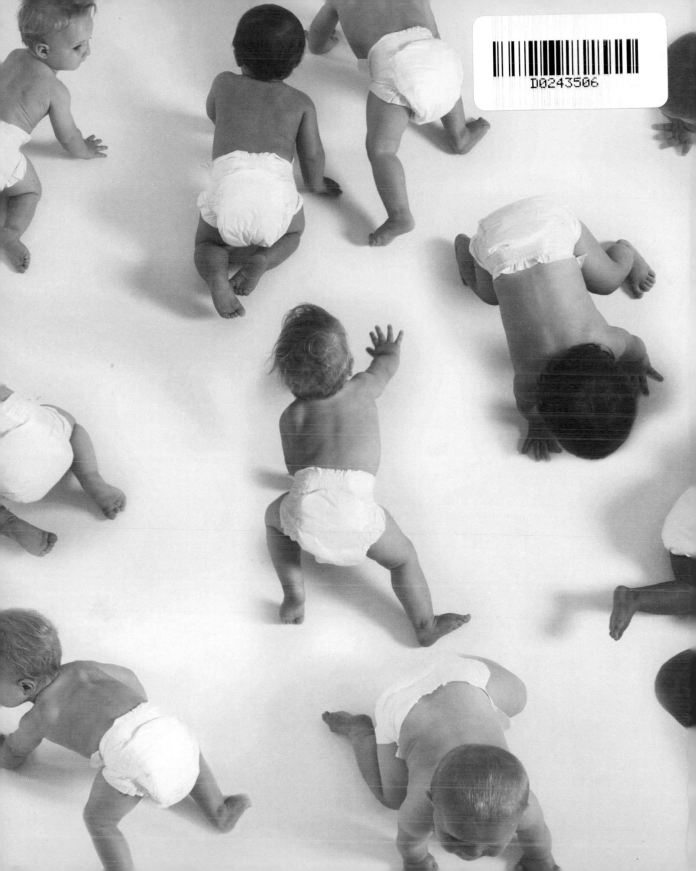